DATE DUE

~~JAN 0 4 2016~~			
NOV 1 4 2016			
NOV 1 3 2017			
NOV 1 2 2018			

Demco, Inc. 38-293

A Patient's Guide to Medical Imaging

A PATIENT'S GUIDE TO
MEDICAL IMAGING

RONALD L. EISENBERG, MD, JD, FACR
Department of Radiology
Beth Israel Deaconess Medical Center
Harvard Medical School
Boston, MA

ALEXANDER R. MARGULIS, MD,
   DSc (hc mult), FACR
Department of Radiology
New York-Presbyterian Hospital
Weill Cornell Medical College
New York, NY

OXFORD
UNIVERSITY PRESS

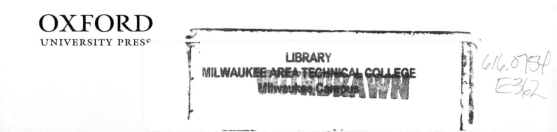

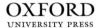

OXFORD
UNIVERSITY PRESS

Oxford University Press, Inc., publishes works that further
Oxford University's objective of excellence
in research, scholarship, and education.

Oxford   New York
Auckland   Cape Town   Dar es Salaam   Hong Kong   Karachi
Kuala Lumpur   Madrid   Melbourne   Mexico City   Nairobi
New Delhi   Shanghai   Taipei   Toronto

With offices in
Argentina   Austria   Brazil   Chile   Czech Republic   France   Greece
Guatemala   Hungary   Italy   Japan   Poland   Portugal   Singapore
South Korea   Switzerland   Thailand   Turkey   Ukraine   Vietnam

Copyright © 2011 by Oxford University Press, Inc.

Published by Oxford University Press, Inc.
198 Madison Avenue, New York, New York 10016

www.oup.com

Library of Congress Cataloging-in-Publication Data

Eisenberg, Ronald L.
  A patient's guide to medical imaging/Ronald L. Eisenberg, Alexander R. Margulis.
    p. cm.
  Includes index.
  ISBN 978-0-19-972991-3
  1. Diagnostic imaging—Popular works. 2. Radiology, Medical—Popular works.
I. Margulis, Alexander R. II. Title.
  RC78.7.D53E375 2011
  616.07'54—dc22   2010020385

9 8 7 6 5 4 3 2 1
Printed in the United States of America
on acid-free paper

To Zina, Avlana, and Cherina

and

To Hedi and Peter

Foreword

In their remarkable new book, *A Patient's Guide to Medical Imaging*, Drs. Ronald L. Eisenberg and Alexander R. Margulis do an outstanding job of presenting the key conceptual and factual information that underlie the practice of medical imaging. They make these concepts and facts understandable and accessible for the lay public.

A Patient's Guide to Medical Imaging is an especially timely and important work because medical imaging plays a central role in the contemporary delivery of health care. As described systematically in this book, imaging plays four important roles—the detection and diagnosis of disease and injury, assessment of response to therapy, screening for early disease in otherwise healthy people, and as an aid to physicians undertaking certain procedures such as biopsies and angioplasties.

In a wide variety of situations, such as suspected stroke or cancer or following trauma, performing an imaging examination is often the fastest and most accurate way of arriving at the correct diagnosis and localization of disease so that the optimal therapy can be applied. *A Patient's Guide to Medical Imaging* will help patients better understand this process and how imaging examinations are vital in helping guide their physicians to the correct diagnostic and therapeutic decisions for them.

The organization of *A Patient's Guide to Medical Imaging* insures that readers will be able to find material of interest quickly and efficiently. After a brief and interesting presentation of the history of medical imaging, each subsequent chapter highlights an important imaging method or area of application. Readers can follow the evolution of the field of medical imaging from its origins in simple x-ray procedures and then on to more complex and technically sophisticated procedures including angiography, ultrasound (US), computed tomography (CT), and magnetic resonance imaging (MRI).

Each chapter follows a common format so that readers can go from chapter to chapter and immediately find the information being sought.

Patients can learn the most important reasons that lead physicians to recommend each imaging method and what to expect if they must undergo an examination themselves. Frequently asked questions are answered, such as "What kind of preparation is required?", "Will I need to fast overnight?", and "What will I feel during the test?"

A particular strength of *A Patient's Guide to Medical Imaging* is the discussion of risks and benefits for each method. Imaging studies are placed in perspective so that patients can understand their strengths and weaknesses. Being able to access this information is invaluable for patients and others involved in their care because decisions must be made to either undergo recommended imaging procedures or not. By being better informed, patients are more able to take an active role in helping make these decisions about their own care and in helping family members and others close to them understand the role that imaging is playing.

Drs. Eisenberg and Margulis are to be congratulated for their invaluable contribution to the better understanding of medical imaging on behalf of patients. The heavy reliance of contemporary medical practice on imaging methods to detect disease and injury and to guide therapy makes *A Patient's Guide to Medical Imaging* a truly important resource.

There are numerous books available aimed at educating the lay public about health care issues. Many of these touch on medical imaging but Dr. Eisenberg and Dr. Margulis's book is the first truly comprehensive work dedicated solely to medical imaging. *A Patient's Guide to Medical Imaging* deserves a place in the library of anyone interested in having access to authoritative information on this topic.

James H. Thrall, MD
Radiologist-in-Chief
Massachusetts General Hospital
Juan M. Taveras Professor of Radiology
Harvard Medical School
Boston, MA

Preface

Imaging has become an indispensable tool in modern medicine, with about 400 million studies performed in the United States each year. In addition to being an essential part of the diagnostic process, medical imaging facilitates follow-up after medical and surgical therapy and provides an alternative to operative intervention. Yet the multiplicity of modalities and techniques used in modern medical imaging may appear as mysterious tests that are greatly confusing and even threatening.

Knowing what to expect can substantially decrease the anxiety associated with medical imaging procedures. Consequently, *A Patient's Guide to Medical Imaging* describes in simple language what the reader needs to know about a wide spectrum of diagnostic procedures, including conventional radiography and commonly performed fluoroscopic (barium) examinations, ultrasound, computed tomography (CT), magnetic resonance imaging (MRI), mammography, nuclear medicine scanning, and angiography. For each of these examinations, *A Patient's Guide to Medical Imaging* provides a general description of the medical indications for the study, the preparation required, a picture of the equipment, an explanation of the sensations one should expect (such as the noise and possible feeling of claustrophobia in the MR scanner, with suggestions on how to prevent it; the movement of the table in the CT scanner; and the application of gel to the skin with ultrasound), about how long the procedure takes to perform and its approximate cost, and its advantages and disadvantages relative to other imaging studies. There is a discussion of the injection and/or ingestion of contrast material, including indications and contraindications, possible allergies, and the need to alert the physicians and staff at the imaging center of prior adverse reactions. This book also describes a wide variety of the currently available image-guided interventional procedures, their indications and risks, and how they compare with surgical alternatives.

A Patient's Guide to Medical Imaging also includes an account of Roentgen's discovery of the x-ray and an overview of the radiologic imaging process and the role of the personnel involved in it. It also addresses such topical issues as radiation exposure, which may make some people reluctant to undergo valuable CT studies and mammography, and health care reform.

We hope that this book will provide a basic understanding of the imaging process and alleviate as much as possible the natural fear of the unknown when preparing to undergo a radiological examination or procedure.

Ronald L. Eisenberg
Alexander R. Margulis

Acknowledgments

We gratefully list the names of those who contributed the many images included in this book:

Memorial Sloan Kettering Cancer Center (New York)
Dr. David Dershaw
Dr. Hedvig Hricak
Dr. Carol Lee
Dr. Elizabeth Morris

Weill Cornell Medical College (New York)
Dr. David A Boyajian
Dr. Stanley J Goldsmith
Dr. Arzu Kovalnikaya
Dr. Kevin Mennit
Dr. Martin Prince
Dr. William Rubenstein
Dr. Pina Sanelli
Dr. Neda Yagan

Siemens Healthcare
Mr. Axel Lorz

Beth Israel Deaconess Medical Center (Boston)
Dr. Muneeb Ahmed
Dr. Neely Hines
Dr. Atif Khan
Mr. Michael Larson
Dr. Diana Litmanovich
Dr. Arra Suresh Reddy

Dr. Janneth Romero
Dr. Priscilla Slanetz
Dr. Jim Wu
Dr. Corrie Yablon

Sharp Hospital (*San Diego*)
Dr. Russell Low

Contents

A Patient's Guide to Medical Imaging

1

INTRODUCTION

Roentgen and His Discovery

Where Did It All Begin?

It was late afternoon on Friday, November 8, 1895. Working alone in his laboratory at the University of Wurzburg in Germany, Wilhelm Conrad Roentgen (Figs. 1-1, 1-2) was performing an experiment, passing charges through a cathode ray tube. Suddenly, in the darkened room he noted a faint flickering glow shimmering on a small bench nearby. Excitedly, Roentgen lit a match and to his great surprise discovered that the source of the mysterious light was a fluorescent barium platinocyanide screen lying on the bench several feet away. He repeated the experiment again and again, continually moving the little screen farther away from the tube and far beyond the range of the cathode rays he was studying. Each time the result was the same, and the glow persisted even when the painted surface of the fluorescent screen was turned in the opposite direction. Whatever it was, the material was able to pass through the lightproof cardboard box he had placed around the tube. When he held a series of objects between the tube and the screen, there was little change in the intensity of the glowing screen. Only lead and platinum seemed to obstruct the ray completely. As he held various materials between the tube and the fluorescent screen, Roentgen was amazed to see the ghostly shadow of the bones and soft tissues of his own fingers. The flesh was transparent, and the bones were fairly opaque. Roentgen concluded that this was a new form of light, which was invisible to the eye and had never been observed or recorded. Thus *x-rays* were discovered, and the field of radiology and medical imaging was born.

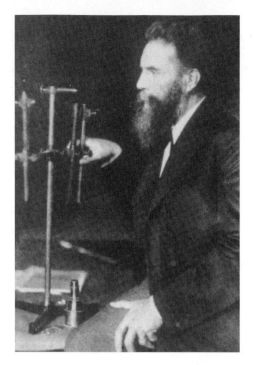

Figure 1-1. Wilhelm Conrad Roentgen. Photograph taken in 1906 while he was Director of the Institute of Physics at the University of Munich.

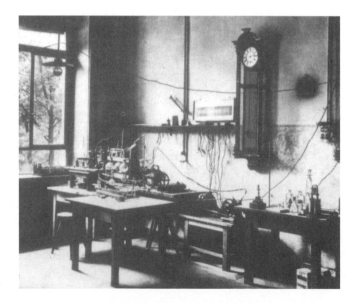

Figure 1-2. Interior of Roentgen's laboratory at Wurzburg.

For the next 7 weeks Roentgen remained secluded in his laboratory, experimenting with this new ray. He asked for his meals to be served in the laboratory and even had his bed moved there so that he could remain undisturbed day and night to pursue any new ideas that might come to him. He constructed a sheet metal cabinet about 7 feet high to produce a permanently dark room. Roentgen added a lead plate to the wall between him and the tube, fortuitously protecting himself from the yet unknown harmful effects of radiation. One evening, Roentgen persuaded his wife to be the subject of an experiment. He placed her hand on a cassette loaded with a photographic plate and made an exposure for 15 minutes. On the developed plate, the bones of her hand appeared light within the darker shadow of the surrounding flesh (Fig. 1-3). Two rings on her finger had almost completely stopped the rays and were clearly visible. His wife shuddered when seeing her skeleton, an experience that she described as a vague premonition of death.

Roentgen's discovery was a sensation, and news of it spread rapidly around the world and sparked public imagination. No longer an obscure university professor, Roentgen became an internationally known scientist. In 1901, Wilhelm Conrad Roentgen was awarded the first Nobel Prize for Physics.

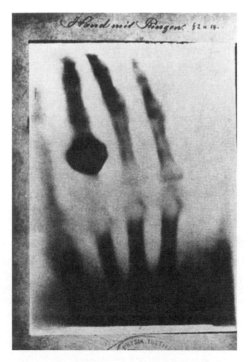

Figure 1-3. First x-ray photograph of Mrs. Roentgen's hand.

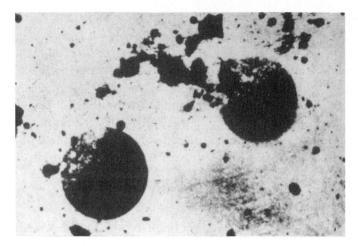

Figure 1-4. First x-ray shadow picture, taken by Arthur W. Goodspeed.

The first x-ray picture

The first x-ray picture was actually produced almost 6 years before Roentgen's discovery. While experimenting with cathode ray tubes, on February 22, 1890, Professor Arthur Goodspeed at the University of Pennsylvania stacked several unexposed photographic plates, on top of which were two coins representing his fare for the Woodland Avenue trolley. When the plates were later developed, some were mysteriously fogged and one contained two dark round disks (Fig. 1-4). Unable to explain the curious shadowgraph, Goodspeed filed them away and they were forgotten until he learned of Roentgen's discovery.

What are x-rays?

X-rays are a form of electromagnetic radiation with much higher energy than visible light. For medical imaging, x-rays are generated by a vacuum tube that uses a high voltage to accelerate the electrons released by a hot cathode to a high velocity. The collision of high-velocity electrons with a metal target, the anode, creates the x-rays. The target in most x-ray tubes is tungsten, though a molybdenum target is used to produce the lower-energy x-rays for mammography.

Overview of the Radiologic Imaging Process

There are many different types of radiologic imaging examinations, ranging from plain radiographs of the chest and bones to newer sophisticated procedures such as ultrasound, computed tomography (CT), and magnetic resonance imaging (MRI). Nevertheless, the basic steps you will experience during the process are similar.

Referral/Scheduling

When you visit your physician, he or she will consider your symptoms, perform an appropriate physical examination, and arrive at a differential diagnosis of possible conditions that could be causing your problem. In many cases, your physician will decide that a particular radiologic imaging study would be helpful in making a specific diagnosis. For example, if you have symptoms of fever, cough, and an elevated white blood cell count suggesting pneumonia, your physician may order a plain chest radiograph. If you are an athlete who has severe shoulder pain from a sports-related injury, an MRI scan of that area may be ordered to detect a muscle or tendon abnormality. If you are pregnant, an obstetric ultrasound scan may be ordered to make certain that your unborn child is developing normally.

If a radiologic imaging procedure is ordered by your physician, you will need to make an appointment to have the examination performed, either at an imaging center or at a hospital-based radiology department. Your physician may recommend a radiology facility or you can go to one of your own choosing, though it may have to be within your health plan's network In many cases, your physician's office staff will help you schedule an appointment.

Examination Preparation

For some imaging examinations, you may be asked to refrain from eating or drinking for a specific amount of time before your appointment. If you have had x-rays and other medical imaging examinations elsewhere that are relevant to your scheduled examination, you may be asked to bring the images or have them sent so that the radiologist can compare the findings.

Generally, you should come for your imaging examination wearing comfortable clothing. For many studies, you will be asked to change into a lightweight medical gown. Before the examination, you may be asked to remove metallic objects such as jewelry, eyeglasses, hairpins, and removable dentures if these could obscure the images. Always remember to bring your insurance card or medical plan information.

Reception

When you arrive at the imaging center or hospital-based imaging department, you will first go to the reception area. Someone will greet you and take your name and other information concerning your health plan or insurance. Usually, you will stay for several minutes in the waiting room before being taken to a dressing area. If your scheduled study allows you to wear your own clothes, you generally will be taken directly to the room where the imaging examination will be performed.

Education

Many radiology facilities have printed material about the type of examination that you are to undergo. This ranges from a single sheet describing the procedure to a full-color illustrated booklet. If specific preparations are required for the test, you should receive explanatory material either from the radiology facility or from the office of the ordering physician. Some imaging centers will ask you to watch a short instructional video about the procedure before your examination. This video may include information about the purpose of the test, its benefits and potential risks, whether any contrast material will have to be injected, and the approximate length of the study. For more complicated examinations, a radiologist may speak with you to explain the procedure in more detail and get an informed consent (see p. 212).

Depending on the type of diagnostic imaging examination, you may be asked a variety of questions relating to allergies, previous surgery, or the presence of metallic devices in your body (e.g., a pacemaker or an artificial joint replacement). A woman of childbearing age should always be asked if she is or might be pregnant.

The Examination Itself

During your examination, it is important that you pay attention to all instructions. Feel free to ask questions if you do not understand what to do. When images are being obtained, you will be asked to remain as still as possible and to hold your breath. It is important for you to remain as calm and relaxed as possible. If you feel anxious or afraid, tell the technologist or radiologist who is performing the examination. Remember that your comfort and safety are always of paramount importance to everyone working in the radiology facility.

Depending on the type of examination, you may be asked to drink barium (which resembles a chalky milkshake), receive a barium enema, or have contrast material (sometimes called *dye*) injected into a vein or artery. Please see the chapter dealing with the specific study you are to have for more details.

After the Examination

Once the diagnostic imaging examination has been performed, you will have a short wait while the technologist and radiologist determine if the images have completely demonstrated the area in question and are of adequate technical quality. In some cases, it may be necessary to repeat part of the examination or to do another imaging test to gain important additional information to help make the diagnosis.

After most imaging studies, you may return to your normal activities. If you have been fasting in preparation for the examination, you can resume your usual diet. Invasive procedures may require a somewhat longer recovery period. If you have been given a sedative to relax as part of the procedure, you will need to have someone else drive you home.

Interpreting the Examination

The imaging examination will be read by a radiologist, a medical doctor who is specially trained to interpret it. At times, the radiologist may speak with you about the results of the study. In most cases, however, the radiologist will dictate an official report that will be sent directly to your primary care or specialist physician, who will then discuss the results with you. In most cases, the completed report is sent to your doctor in 1–2 days. Your doctor can indicate on the request form if there is a medical need for a faster report.

Radiology Personnel

Radiologist

The diagnostic radiologist is a physician who has extensive specialized training in interpreting medical images. These include plain radiographs, fluoroscopic studies, ultrasound, CT, MRI, nuclear medicine, and interventional procedures.

Becoming a radiologist requires at least 13 years of training following high school. After 4 years of college, the future radiologist becomes a doctor by completing 4 years of medical school. This is followed by a year of internship and 4 years of residency, which are required to become a general radiologist. Most radiologists then spend 1 or 2 additional years doing extensive clinical work and related research to become a subspecialist in the imaging of either one organ system (e.g., the breast, chest, abdomen, musculoskeletal system, neurologic system) or one imaging modality (e.g., CT, MRI, ultrasound, nuclear medicine).

Radiologists usually are board certified, meaning that they have taken and passed a series of comprehensive examinations indicating that they have the level of knowledge, skill, and understanding essential to the practice of their specialty. They also must earn yearly Continuing Medical Education credits and take a recertification examination every 10 years. Consequently, you should make certain that all the radiologists at the imaging facility where you are having your examination are board certified.

Radiologic Technologist

Radiologic technologists operate the radiographic equipment to produce images. They are responsible for proper positioning of the patient and for adjusting exposure controls to obtain optimal images while using protective devices to minimize radiation. Becoming a radiologic technologist requires a formal 2-year training program for a certificate or associate degree or a 4-year bachelor's degree. Many technologists elect additional training to become eligible to work with highly specialized equipment such as ultrasound, CT, and MRI.

Most radiologic technologists take a certification examination that tests their knowledge and cognitive skills and ensures that they have met the required educational preparation and ethics standards. To maintain this initial registration and be designated as a registered technologist) (RT), the technologist must take continuing education courses. Therefore, you should always make certain that the imaging facility where you are having your radiology examination employs only fully registered technologists.

Radiologist Assistant

A radiologist assistant is an experienced registered technologist who has received additional training and works under the close supervision of a radiologist to perform and assist with advanced tasks. These tasks include involvement in patient care and evaluation, assessing image quality, assisting the radiologist with invasive procedures, and directly performing selected fluoroscopic procedures such as barium studies. However, only the responsible radiologist may dictate an official written interpretation of the study findings.

Radiology Nurse

Some radiology facilities employ registered nurses to provide care and support to patients during imaging procedures. They work primarily in interventional radiology, where they monitor vital signs, administer contrast material and medications, and offer postprocedure care under the supervision of a radiologist.

Radiology Scheduler/Receptionist

The often overlapping duties of this individual include online and telephone scheduling of patients for examinations, determining the diagnosis code, ensuring that preauthorization requirements have been completed, explaining the preparation required for each examination, and confirming appointment times of imaging studies.

Radiology Transcriptionist

Radiology transcriptionists are responsible for typing the official interpretations of imaging studies that are dictated by the radiologist. In addition to requiring typing skills, they must have knowledge of medical terminology, including words specifically used in radiology.

These highly specialized and valued individuals are rapidly disappearing from the scene, as voice recognition systems are increasingly displacing typed reports with ones that are generated by a computer. This adds speed and is incorporated in picture archiving and communicating systems (PACS).

Radiation Exposure

Many people have an irrational fear of radiation and are seriously concerned when their physician recommends an x-ray imaging procedure. In most cases, the diagnostic or therapeutic benefit of the x-ray examination far outweighs any potential risk. Nevertheless, it is important to understand the effects of radiation on the body and the ways in which to decrease exposure.

According to a study by the National Council on Radiation Protection and Measurements (2009), there has been a sevenfold increase in the exposure of Americans to ionizing radiation in the past 20 years. Medical imaging is now the second leading source of radiation exposure in the United States, responsible for almost 50% compared to only 20% two decades earlier.

Most of this increased medical exposure relates to CT and nuclear medicine examinations (Fig. 1-5).

It may come as a surprise that a large proportion of this increase in radiation exposure is not related to x-ray studies performed by radiologists. The major cause of the increase is *self-referral* studies performed in the offices of nonradiologists. As noted in a 2008 report from the Government Accountability Office, during the previous two decades the increase in charges to Medicare for CT, MRI, and nuclear medicine examinations performed in nonradiologist physicians' offices increased three times as rapidly as the rate of charges for the same examinations performed in hospitals and independent imaging facilities run by radiologists. More troubling, a study by Blue Cross Blue Shield suggested that nearly half of these examinations may have been unnecessary. This means that a large percentage of the increasing exposure to medical x-rays cannot be justified on the grounds of benefit to the patient.

Radiation Damage to Living Tissue

During a radiographic examination, a fraction of the high-energy x-rays pass through the body to produce the image. Many x-ray photons are absorbed by tissue within the body. The transfer of energy causes the ionization (excitation) of atoms and molecules within cellular structures, which can result in the production of free radicals, the breaking of chemical bonds and the production of new chemical bonds and cross-linkage between large molecules, and damage to molecules such as DNA, RNA, and proteins that regulate vital processes in the cells. At low doses of x-rays, such as those received every day from natural background radiation, most cellular damage is rapidly repaired. However, some might be permanent. High radiation doses, such as those suffered by the victims of the atomic bomb blasts at Hiroshima and Nagasaki at the end of World War II, are far higher than those used in any imaging procedures and cause extensive cell death. In such cases, the body cannot replace cells fast enough, leading to failure of organs to function properly. Some researchers have attempted to extrapolate the damage due to radiation from nuclear bomb explosions downward to doses from x-ray imaging examinations, but their findings are highly controversial.

Various tissues in the body differ in their sensitivity to radiation. As a general rule, the most sensitive tissues are those with cells that divide rapidly and are relatively nonspecialized (blood-forming organs, skin, gastrointestinal tract). The most differentiated tissues, such as the nervous system, are least sensitive to radiation. That explains why the developing fetus is more sensitive to radiation during early pregnancy (first trimester) than in

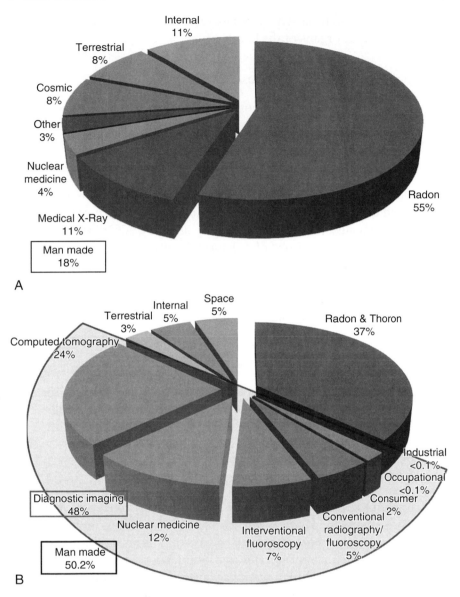

Figure 1-5. Exposure sources for collective effective dose to residents of the United States. (A) 1982, (B) 2006. Note the dramatic increase in the percentage of radiation exposure from diagnostic imaging (15% to 48%). (National Council on Radiation Protection and Measurements)

the late stages (third trimester), when there has been progressive differentiation in the various organs of the body.

Early and Late Effects of High Doses of Radiation

The harmful effects of radiation on the body can be divided according to when they appear. High doses of radiation rapidly delivered to the entire body of a healthy adult, such as from nuclear bombs or rare nuclear plant accidents such as Chernobyl, can cause acute radiation sickness. This potentially fatal condition is characterized by bone marrow destruction and decreased production of blood cells, injury to the gastrointestinal tract with nausea and diarrhea, and generalized fatigue. Irradiation of only a part of the body may cause hair loss and burning or mere reddening of the skin. Delayed effects of high doses of radiation usually appear months or years after exposure. Cataracts may develop after irradiation of the lens of the eye. There is also an increased risk of leukemia, multiple myeloma, and cancers of the breast, lung, thyroid, and skin developing as late as 10 years or more following high-dose radiation exposure.

Measurement of Radiation Exposure

The scientific unit of measurement for radiation dose was long calculated in terms of millirem (mrem). More recently, the term used is the millisievert (mSv), named for a Swedish physicist.

    1 mrem = 10 mSv
    100 mrem = 1 mSv

The current baseline risk of cancer induction in the United States is about 25%. By extrapolating downward from radiation damage related to the nuclear explosions at Hiroshima and Nagasaki, it has been estimated that a dose of 10 mrem (0.1 mSv) creates a risk of death from cancer of approximately 1 in 1,000,000. Many scientists are disputing even this low figure, considering it arbitrary and based on false assumptions.

Table 1-1 presents the dosages of some major radiographic examinations.

Risk to Health of Low Doses of Radiation

The risk of low-level radiation, such as that used in diagnostic imaging, is not known. There is scientific evidence that doses greater than 100–200 mSv have a significant association with the risk of developing cancer. Most experts believe that the risk from lower doses, as from infrequent CT or

Table 1-1 Dosages of Major Radiographic Examinations

Examination	Average Effective Dosage (mSv)
Chest radiograph	
Frontal	0.02
Lateral	0.04
Thoracic spine radiograph	
Frontal	0.4
Lateral	0.3
Lumbar spine radiograph	
Frontal	0.7
Lateral	0.3
Abdomen or pelvis radiograph (frontal)	0.7
Nuclear medicine lung scan	2
CT (head)	2
CT (chest)	8
CT (abdomen or pelvis)	10
CT (cardiac)	18–22

other imaging examinations, is very small, and there are no data showing that medical imaging actually causes cancer. It is extremely difficult to estimate the risk of causing cancer, because most of the radiation exposure received from medical imaging studies is close to background levels. At these low doses, the risk of radiation-induced cancers is so low that, even if it exists, it cannot be easily distinguished from normal levels of cancer occurrence. In addition, leukemia or solid tumors induced by radiation are indistinguishable from those that result from other causes. Yet it must be remembered that the dose of medical radiation may be cumulative over a lifetime, and x-rays have been officially classified as *potential carcinogens.*

In most cases, the risk associated with medical x-ray imaging is similar to, or even smaller than, that encountered in everyday activities or occupations that are considered safe. Nevertheless, it is reasonable to assume that any radiation exposure, no matter how small, carries some risk. Therefore, it is important that any unnecessary radiation be avoided. The benefits of a radiographic procedure must always outweigh the risks. A popular acronym expressing one approach to minimize the radiation risk is to keep the dose ALARA—"As Low As Reasonably Achievable."

The small lifetime risk of cancer depends on several factors. It is higher for x-rays received at an earlier age and increases as a person undergoes more x-ray exams and the accumulated radiation dose gets higher.

Women may have a somewhat higher lifetime risk than men of developing cancer from radiation after receiving the same exposures at the same ages.

The decision regarding whether to have an x-ray examination is based on the specific medical situation, based on the diagnostic or therapeutic benefit weighed against any potential risk from radiation. For low-dose examinations such as plain radiographs, there is usually no question. For higher-dose studies, especially CT, frequent previous examinations could be a consideration because of the cumulative effect of radiation exposure. Imaging procedures that do not use ionizing radiation, such as ultrasound and MRI, may be an alternative. However, even with higher-dose studies, it is very likely that the benefit of an x-ray examination easily outweighs any possible risk from radiation.

It is important to remember that x-rays are produced only when the equipment is momentarily turned on for the exposure. As with visible light, no radiation remains after the equipment is turned off.

Genetic Effects of Radiation

Genetic effects are those that appear in the descendants of a person exposed to x-rays as a result of radiation damage to the reproductive cells. In humans, there is no direct evidence of radiation-induced genetic effects even at high doses. Even if there is some effect, it is much less than the other risks associated with radiation and is easily outweighed by the benefits gained from appropriate imaging studies. Therefore, the techniques used to protect the exposed person from harm are also effective in protecting future generations. However, for examinations of children and of adults of reproductive age, the gonads (ovaries of women and testicles of men) must be shielded from radiation, usually with a lead apron.

Naturally Occurring Background Radiation

Every person is constantly exposed to ionizing radiation from natural sources, which is known as *background radiation*. There are three major sources of background radiation:

- Radioactive substances in the Earth's crust (especially naturally occurring isotopes of uranium and thorium and their decay products, such as the gas radon); these isotopes, which were part of the Earth when it formed 4 billion years ago, have extremely long half-lives (100 million years or more).
- Cosmic rays (extremely high-energy particles, primarily protons, that bombard the Earth from outer space); because the Earth's atmosphere

acts as a shield, the exposure to cosmic rays is greater at higher elevations (e.g., about twice as much in Denver as at sea level).

• Trace amounts of radioactivity in the body (primarily from naturally radioactive materials from the food we eat and the air we breathe, including tritium (hydrogen 3, carbon-14, and potassium-40).

The average person in the United States receives a radiation dose of about 3 mSv per year from naturally occurring radioactive materials and cosmic radiation from outer space. The added dose from cosmic rays on a commercial airplane flight from coast to coast is about 0.03 mSv. Although the altitude of the place where one lives is an important factor in overall exposure, the largest source of background radiation is radon gas in the home (about 2 mSv per year). Like other sources of background radiation, this varies widely from one part of the country to another.

An interesting approach is to compare the radiation dose related to a specific radiographic study to natural background radiation. For example, the radiation exposure from one chest x-ray is equivalent to that received from our natural surroundings in about 10 days. The numbers for some other common imaging studies are presented in Table 1-2.

CT and Radiation Exposure

The development of CT in the 1980s revolutionized medical imaging, dramatically improving the ability of radiologists to make accurate diagnoses. The use of CT has skyrocketed, from about 3 million examinations in 1980 to more than 65 million in 2005. In the United States, more than 150,000 CT studies are performed each day. This represents about a quarter of the examinations performed worldwide and is equivalent to one CT examination for every 4.5 Americans.

Table 1-2 Background Radiation Equivalents of Radiographic Studies

Procedure	Background radiation
Bone densitometry (DEXA)	1 day
Mammography	3 months
Hysterosalpingography	4 months
Spine radiograph	6 months
Upper gastrointestinal series	8 months
Barium enema	16 months
CTomputed (head)	8 months
CT (chest or abdomen)	3 years

The increase in CT examinations is related to the development of multi-detector scanners, which can provide exquisitely detailed anatomic studies in a few seconds. The images can be postprocessed to give frontal (coronal) or lateral (sagittal) views. However, this comes at the cost of a huge increase in radiation exposure, since hundreds of individual x-ray scans are obtained during the procedure. Sophisticated CT scans of the abdomen or chest are associated with a radiation dose 50–100 times that of a two-view plain chest radiograph.

Manufacturers of CT equipment and radiologists are working together to reduce the radiation dose as much as possible without jeopardizing diagnostic quality. For example, studies have shown that images obtained by reducing the current within the x-ray tube can decrease exposure by up to 50% without reducing the detectability of known abnormalities such as pulmonary nodules or pulmonary emboli. Limiting a CT study to the area of diagnostic concern makes it possible to take fewer individual slices, thus reducing the radiation exposure. In many cases, it is possible to eliminate the precontrast CT scan and to obtain images only after contrast material has been injected, effectively decreasing the radiation dose by half. Repeat CT scans to follow up a patient with lung nodules or after interventional procedures (biopsy or drainage) can be performed successfully with much lower radiation doses to the patient. Shielding devices are now available to dramatically reduce radiation exposure to the breast during cardiac CT imaging.

An important part of radiologists' training is to develop awareness of imaging alternatives that do not use x-rays. Therefore, the radiologist may suggest to your physician an alternative study, such as ultrasound or MRI, that can provide similar diagnostic information without any radiation exposure. The American College of Radiology has added a column on "relative radiation level" to its guidelines on the appropriateness of various imaging procedures for specific clinical situations so that radiologists and referring clinicians alike are made aware of the differences in radiation exposure among these alternatives.

Interventional Procedures and Radiation Exposure

The dose of radiation from an interventional radiology procedure depends on the imaging technique used to guide the examination. Some procedures can be performed under ultrasound guidance, which uses no x-rays and has no known risk. Others can be performed using MRI, which also does not use ionizing radiation but cannot be done in patients with implanted pacemakers, defibrillators, and some other metallic devices.

Many interventional procedures are performed under fluoroscopic or CT guidance, both of which entail the use of x-rays. The amount of radiation exposure varies widely, depending on the complexity of the procedure, but usually the associated risk of developing a cancer is not a major concern when compared to the benefits. Some of these procedures are literally life-saving or avoid the need for extensive complicated surgery, general anesthesia, and prolonged hospitalization.

Pregnancy and Radiation

The developing fetus, especially during the first 20 weeks, has a large number of rapidly developing cells and thus is especially sensitive to radiation. Potential effects associated with prenatal radiation exposure include growth retardation, small size of the head or brain, mental retardation, and childhood cancer. Therefore, it is extremely important that a woman scheduled for an x-ray examination inform her physician, the radiologic technologist, or the radiologist that she is or may be pregnant.

The vast majority of diagnostic imaging procedures do not pose a substantial risk to the developing fetus. For example, plain radiographs of the chest and extremities do not directly expose the fetus to any x-rays. Moreover, the technologist will typically wrap the abdomen of a pregnant woman with a lead shield to prevent any radiation exposure.

If it is necessary to examine the abdominal and pelvic structures of a pregnant woman, alternative imaging studies will be seriously considered. Rather than a CT scan of the area, with its relatively high radiation dose, it is highly likely that an ultrasound examination or MRI will be substituted, since neither uses any ionizing radiation or has been shown to pose any substantial risk to a pregnancy.

Nuclear medicine procedures pose a unique risk for the young child who is being breast-fed, since some of the radionuclide passes into the mother's milk. To prevent this possibility, it is important for a nursing mother to inform her physician and the radiologic technologist before the examination begins. In most cases, a nursing mother will be asked to discontinue breast feeding for several days, instead pumping her breasts and discarding the milk.

What Should You Do?

If you are concerned about the risk of radiation, you have the right to ask your health care professional about the benefits of any proposed x-ray examination. It is reasonable to question whether there are other procedures that might provide a good assessment or treatment for your medical condition without any radiation risk. If your health care professional believes that an x-ray examination is medically necessary, remember that the risk of not having the imaging study is generally far greater than the small radiation risk associated with the study. Radiologists make every effort to ensure that the least number of x-ray images are obtained, and technologists take these images at the lowest radiation dose possible. (In addition, a lead apron should be used to cover the reproductive organs in the abdomen when performing an x-ray examination of the chest, and a protective lead shield should be placed over the thyroid gland when dental x-rays are made.) Conversely, do not insist on having an x-ray examination performed if your health care professional explains that there is no need for it.

Always tell the radiologic technologist if you are or may be pregnant. If you or your child is having an x-ray study, ask whether a lead apron or another shield should be used. Keep a record of your x-ray history, including dental x-rays. This should include the date and type of examination, the name of the referring physician, and the facility where the study was performed and the images are stored. Show this card to your health care professional to avoid unnecessary duplication of x-rays of the same body part. Also, it may be extremely important for the radiologist to have access to the images from previous x-ray examinations performed at another facility. Demonstrating no change in the appearance of a suspected abnormality over several years may mean that the finding is of no significance, thus precluding the need for a high-dose CT scan to prove this. When there is a need for x-rays of your teeth, ask whether your dentist uses digital radiography, which provides similar-quality images at a much lower radiation dose.

Cost of Imaging Procedures

Radiologic imaging examinations vary widely in cost. Although less expensive procedures sometimes yield approximately the same results as more costly studies, it is important to realize that adding a more elaborate and expensive test to a relatively inexpensive one will cost the patient more than if the more sophisticated procedure had simply been ordered and performed initially. Moreover, in a hospital setting, making a rapid diagnosis with a more expensive but sophisticated test and promptly instituting appropriate treatment may be cost-effective in terms of improving patient care and decreasing the length of the hospital stay.

It is difficult to give the precise cost of a specific procedure, since there may be substantial difference in charges among various institutions and in different geographic regions. To give you an idea of the relative costs, the charges for the imaging procedures listed in Table 1-3 are expressed as

Table 1-3 Cost of Various Procedures Compared to a Plain Chest Radiograph

Barium enema	2.5x
Upper gastrointestinal series	3x
Hysterosalpingogram	3x
Ultrasound	3x
Radionuclide scan (lung, bone)	3–4x
Echocardiogram	4–5x
CT	7–10x
MRI	8–12x

multiples of the plain chest radiograph (the most frequent radiographic study), which is designated "x."

Some interventional radiographic procedures are quite expensive, but they may be extremely cost-effective because they eliminate the need for surgery or hospitalization and allow the patient to return more quickly to normal activity. For example, using the relative cost system, angiography would be 8–12x, while surgery would be more than 40x.

Your Bill for Radiology Services

The bill you receive for an imaging study may be divided into two categories: technical and professional. The technical fee is the cost of performing the examination. This is related to the expense of purchasing and maintaining the equipment and includes facility overhead for space and utilities as well as salaries for the technical staff, transcriptionists, and other employees. The professional fee is the payment to the radiologist for overseeing/ performing the examination, interpreting the results, making the diagnosis, and dictating a formal report to be sent to your physician. On average, the technical fee constitutes about 80% of the total cost of an imaging study.

Health Care Reform

While there is no question that the United States desperately needed health care reform, being the only developed country in the world with a sizable proportion of its citizens uninsured, it is worrisome that not a single Republican in either the Senate or the House of Representatives voted for it. The other troubling facts are that many meaningful reforms do not start until 2014 and that many of the implementation policies are left to the states, several of which are suing the federal government and calling the law unconstitutional.

It is possible that in future years the law may even be repealed. However, some important benefits are scheduled for immediate implementation:

1. The uninsured are eligible to receive immediate access to coverage through high-risk pools if they are uninsured due to preexisting conditions; children can remain on their parents' plans until they are 26 years of age.
2. Insurance companies are barred from removing coverage when a person becomes ill, denying coverage to children with preexisting conditions, and imposing lifetime coverage caps.
3. Small businesses can receive tax credits to purchase insurance for their employees.
4. Some favorable changes are available for Medicare drug prescription recipients.

In **2013,** Medicare payroll taxes will increase; these increases will also be applied to unearned income for individuals earning more than $200,000 a year and families earning more than $250,000. It is not until **2014** that the most meaningful provisions come into effect:

1. Most citizens are obligated to buy health insurance or pay a penalty. Individuals and small businesses can buy packages through state exchanges.
2. Insurance companies are prohibited from refusing to provide insurance and setting prices on the basis of health status.
3. Businesses with 50 or more employees must provide health insurance or be fined.

In **2018,** a much-resisted provision goes into effect: High-cost employer-provided health insurance beneficiaries ($27,500 for a family, $10,200 for individuals) are subjected to a 40% excise tax.

The two worrisome aspects for the future of the legislation are:

1. With the polarization of Congress and with two forthcoming elections until **2014,** much of this legislation may be amended or even repealed, as was the Medicare Catastrophic Coverage Act of 1988.
2. Much of the implementation of the legislation depends on the states, some of which are ill prepared to execute it, even if they are willing to cooperate. Many states, particularly in the Deep South, are unwilling to put the programs into effect.

Our provisional advice to our readers: Take advantage of whatever is available to you and investigate your local options before using any services.

2

CONVENTIONAL RADIOLOGY

Plain Radiographs

What Is Plain Radiography?

Although there have been dramatic technical advances in medical imaging over the past 40 years, about half of the examinations interpreted by radiologists are plain radiographs. Because of their speed, widespread availability, and relatively low cost, plain radiographs remain the initial imaging procedure to evaluate the lung, heart, and skeleton. Often called *plain x-rays*, they are actually the images produced by x-rays, which cannot be seen by the human eye.

The black-and-white radiographic image is a *photographic negative* of the object being x-rayed. The relative shades represent how much of the x-ray beam is blocked by a specific part of the body. Calcium in bone blocks the passage of all or a very large portion of the x-ray beam, so healthy bones appear white on the outside (cortex) and gray on the inside (medullary cavity). Conversely, air permits almost all of the x-rays to pass through, so a normal lung appears black. Between these extremes are skin, muscle, blood vessels, liver, and spleen, which allow an intermediate number of the x-rays to pass through and appear as various shades of gray (*soft-tissue density*).

Plain radiographs are usually taken by a registered radiologic technologist and then interpreted by a radiologist, who is responsible for describing the imaging findings, making a diagnosis, and recommending any additional imaging procedures that are necessary.

Historical vignette

Plain radiography is the oldest type of x-ray study. It is actually a form of photography, since it is a process whereby images are obtained on sensitized surfaces by the action of light or other radiant energy. Like photography, radiography may use visible light, as emitted from fluorescent screens, or it may use invisible light that differs from visible light only in wavelength. Initially, radiography used photographic emulsions as recording media, first on glass plates and then on acetate-based film. Today plain radiographic images are viewed on computer monitors.

Why Am I Having this Test?

The three major types of plain radiographic examinations are those of the chest, bones, and abdomen.

Your physician may order a chest radiograph if your clinical symptoms suggest such conditions as:

- Pneumonia (Fig. 2-1)
- Emphysema (Fig. 2-2)
- Lung cancer
- Heart failure
- Pulmonary embolism (blood clot blocking an artery to the lungs)
- Pneumothorax (air in the thoracic cavity, especially due to trauma, that may compress the lung and prevent it from fully expanding) (Fig. 2-3)
- Fractured rib (or any bone of the thorax)

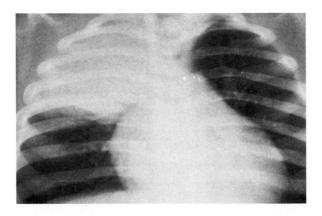

Figure 2-1. Pneumonia. The triangular white area represents a consolidation of the entire right upper lobe.

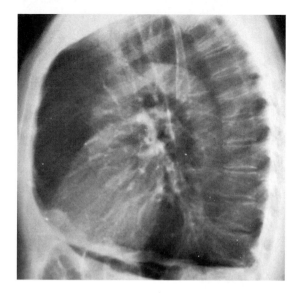

Figure 2-2. Emphysema. Lateral view demonstrates severe overexpansion of the lungs with flattening of the diaphragm. There is also increased size and darkness of the air space behind the sternum and the appearance of a "barrel" chest.

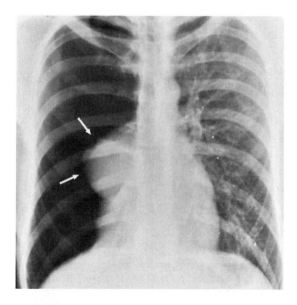

Figure 2-3. Pneumothorax. The right hemithorax is filled with free air and there are no markings within the right lung, which is completely collapsed (arrows).

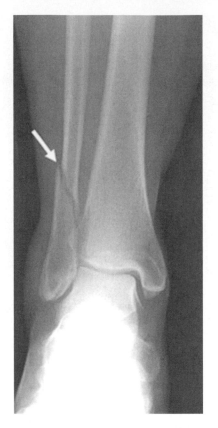

Figure 2-4. Fracture. Frontal view of the ankle shows an oblique fracture of the fibula (arrow).

Your physician may order a bone radiograph if your clinical symptoms suggest such conditions as:

- Fracture of dislocation (trauma) (Fig. 2-4)
- Arthritis (Fig. 2-5)
- Infection of a bone (osteomyelitis) or joint (septic joint)
- Scoliosis (abnormal curvature of the spine)
- Bone tumor
- Follow-up of fracture healing or joint replacement surgery

Your physician may order an abdominal radiograph if your clinical symptoms suggest such conditions as:

- Intestinal obstruction (Fig. 2-6)
- Bowel perforation (Fig. 2-7)
- Stone in the urinary tract (kidneys, ureters, bladder) or gallbladder
- Foreign body (e.g., swallowed coins, bullet fragments)

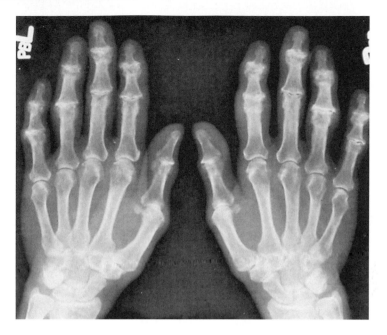

Figure 2-5. Osteoarthritis. Narrowing of all the interphalangeal joints with hypertrophic spurring indicates severe degenerative disease.

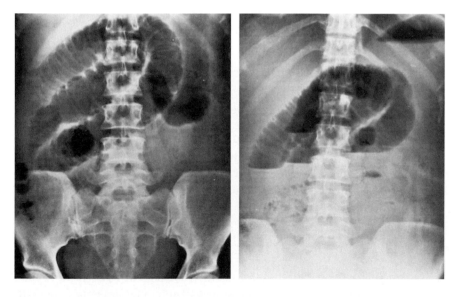

Figure 2-6. Small bowel obstruction. Two views show prominent dilatation of small bowel loops without any gas distally, consistent with a complete obstruction. Characteristic air-fluid levels are seen on the upright image on the right.

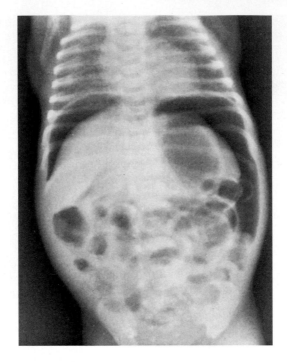

Figure 2-7. Pneumoperitoneum. Large amount of free gas in the peritoneal cavity from an intestinal perforation outlines the top of the liver and, spleen and the underside of the diaphragm.

If you have sciatica or other symptoms of degenerative disc disease, your physician may order a plain radiograph of your spine.

How Do I Prepare for a Plain Radiograph?

Unlike many other imaging studies, plain radiographic examinations do not require any special preparation. Depending on the part of the body being examined, you may be asked to undress and be given a lightweight gown to wear. You also will be asked to remove any jewelry or metal objects that might obscure the x-ray image.

How Is the Test Performed?

If you can stand, chest radiography usually consists of two views (frontal and lateral), with you standing against a wall-mounted cassette (Fig. 2-8). Other plain radiographs may be taken with you lying on an examination table (Fig. 2-9). Pillows or sandbags may be used if you need to be placed

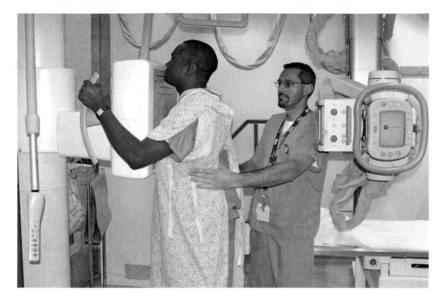

Figure 2-8. Positioning for an upright frontal radiograph of the chest.

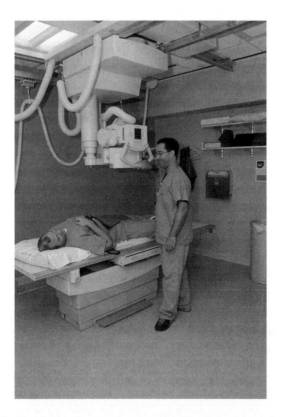

Figure 2-9. Positioning for a supine frontal radiograph of the abdomen.

at an angle for a special view. Once you are positioned correctly, the technologist will move to a shielded control room and expose the image. In most cases, the technologist will watch you through a window of leaded glass. You may be asked to hold your breath for a few seconds as each picture is taken so that the movement of breathing does not blur the image. In most cases, the entire procedure will take less than 15 minutes, though you will only be exposed to radiation for less than 1 second.

If your child is being examined, you usually will be allowed to stay in the room during the test as long as you wear a lead apron to protect you from unnecessary radiation exposure while the images are being made. When the extremity of a child is being examined, at times it may be important to also take a picture of the opposite side for comparison. Restraints or other mobilization devices may be necessary to keep infants and very young children still. This is important, since any sudden movements could blur the image and make it necessary to take a repeat film (with added radiation exposure).

What Will You Feel?

You will not feel anything when the x-ray image is taken. In most cases, the only discomfort you will experience relates to the hardness of the x-ray table. X-ray rooms tend to be kept cool to protect the equipment from overheating, but you will be given a sheet or blanket if requested. Some of the positions required for plain radiographs may be uncomfortable, but you will need to maintain them for only a few seconds. If you have suffered an injury and cannot assume the usual position for the examination, the technologist may be able to take a similar view with you in a more comfortable one.

After the procedure has been completed, you usually can resume your normal activities.

Risks of the Procedure

Plain radiographic examinations are safe procedures. Great care is taken to use the lowest radiation dose needed to produce diagnostic images. Because the developing fetus is especially sensitive to radiation, always tell the technologist if you are or may be pregnant.

Portable Radiographs

In a hospital setting, a seriously ill patient or one confined to bed cannot go to the radiology department for a plain radiographic examination. Examples are patients in an intensive care unit or those undergoing surgical procedures in the operating room. In such cases, a special x-ray machine is taken to the patient to obtain a so-called portable radiograph. Portable radiographs produce electronic images that are entered into the same electronic system used for all other hospital x-ray studies and are interpreted by a radiologist.

Many portable radiographs are exposed with the patient lying on the back (supine) in bed. If possible, portable chest radiographs are obtained with the patient propped up with pillows, with the x-ray tube in front and the cassette placed behind the back. The more upright the patient is positioned, the clearer the resulting image. Portable images of the abdomen are usually obtained with the patient supine.

At times, the patient may be asked to lie on the side, with the cassette placed behind the back and the x-ray tube positioned in front so that the beam is parallel to the bed. This so-called lateral decubitus view is used to evaluate the amount of fluid in the pleural space or to determine whether there is any free air in the abdomen that indicates a perforated bowel.

If at all possible, every effort should be made to obtain all x-ray images in the radiology department, because portable films are generally of poorer quality than those taken with permanent equipment. However, if the patient cannot come to the radiology department, portable images are the best (and only) choice.

Historical vignette

One of the earliest uses of portable radiographs was in a military environment. However, generation of the electric current needed to run the machine was a serious problem. In the River War for control over the valley of the Nile (1896–1898) in Egypt, the solution was to produce electricity by charging wet batteries with a dynamo rigged up to the rear wheel of a tandem bicycle. This required two cyclists, pedaling as hard as they could to overcome the resistance, since the high temperature and humidity prevented any single soldier from cycling for more than 30 minutes at a time.

Marie Curie, the only person to have won two Nobel Prizes (for her discovery of radium and for other work on radioactivity), was much better known in France for her development of the *radiological car* during World War I. These mobile units, which contained x-ray equipment with a dynamo to supply electricity, were affectionately named *little Curies*.

Fluoroscopy

What Is Fluoroscopy?

Fluoroscopy is an imaging technique in which radiologists obtain continuous real-time images of the internal structures of a patient, much like an "x-ray movie." In the first fluoroscopic studies, the part of the body being examined was placed between an x-ray tube and a fluorescent screen. Modern fluoroscopes connect the screen to an x-ray image intensifier, which greatly enhances the detail, and the images are displayed on a television monitor. They also can be recorded by a video camera and stored for later viewing.

Common Examinations Using Fluoroscopy

In the past, fluoroscopy was used alone as a diagnostic procedure, such as to assess the movements of the heart and diaphragm (sniff test). More commonly, fluoroscopy is now used as part of more complex examinations and procedures such as the following:

- Gastrointestinal (GI) studies (barium swallow, upper GI series, barium enema, examinations for postoperative leaks) to follow passage of the contrast material through the alimentary tract
- Cardiac catheterization to demonstrate the flow of iodinated contrast material through the coronary arteries and to determine whether they are narrowed or obstructed
- Arthrography to inject contrast material into a joint
- Insertion of intravenous catheters to guide them to the desired location
- Checking for proper placement of tubes (gastrostomy, jejunostomy, nephrostomy tubes)
- Localizing foreign bodies
- Orthopedic surgery to guide the placement of metallic fixation devices to stabilize fractures

Why Was Fluoroscopy Developed and How Does It Work?

Fluoroscopy dates back to the discovery of x-rays by Roentgen in 1895, when he observed a glow of light coming from a nearby barium platinocyanide screen in his laboratory. Within months of this discovery, the first medical fluoroscopes were created. These homemade devices permitted direct observation of an object, such as a hand, rather than imaging it on a photographic plate. They consisted of a tube with a fluorescent screen on one end and an opening for the eyes at the other (Fig. 2-10). If x-rays were present, the screen would glow with characteristic fluorescence. An opaque substance placed between the x-ray source and the fluorescent screen would produce a dark shadow. Unlike a photographic plate, there was no permanent shadow left on the screen. As soon as the generation of x-rays ceased, the crystals in the screen stopped fluorescing and the screen became dark.

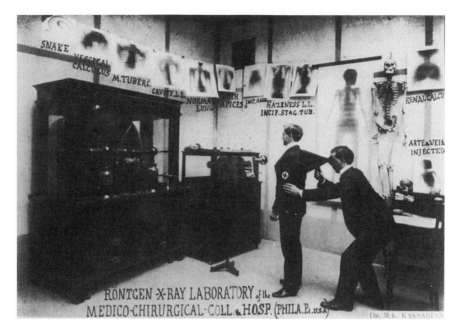

Figure 2-10. Early fluoroscopic examination at the Kassabian Clinic in Philadelphia. The patient is positioned between the open x-ray source (left) and the physician with bent knee holding a hand-held fluoroscopy device.

The first commercially available fluoroscopes used screens made of calcium tungstate, which Thomas Edison showed produced the brightest images of more than 8000 substances he tested. Edison was so elated with his new screen that he incorrectly predicted that the moving images from fluoroscopy would completely replace still x-ray photographs.

Early fluoroscopy was beset with important problems. Because of the low levels of light produced, operators were required to sit in the darkened procedure room for up to a half hour to accustom their eyes to the low light before beginning an examination. Red goggles were developed to address this problem of dark adaptation. However, serious problems remained. Spending hours peering at a dimly fluorescing screen caused significant eyestrain, and prolonged exposure to radiation from unshielded x-ray tubes often led to serious injury.

The development of the x-ray image intensifier and the television camera in the 1950s completely revolutionized the use of fluoroscopy in clinical diagnosis. Image intensifiers permitted the light produced by the fluoroscopic screen to be dramatically amplified so that images could be seen even in a lighted room without prior dark adaptation. The addition of the television camera made it possible to see the images on a remote monitor so

Historical vignette

Ignorance of the harmful effects of x-rays led to trivial uses of fluoroscopy that are no longer permitted. In the 1930s, when shoe stores began to feature x-ray photographs of feet cramped by poorly fitting shoes, shoe-fitting fluoroscopes soon became commercially available (Fig. 2-11). These devices had an opening at the bottom for the customer's feet (often those of a child) and three viewing openings so that the customer, the sales clerk, and one other person could observe the screen. Most of these devices were equipped with a push-button timer, which generally was set for 20 seconds. However, since repeated exposures could be made by simply releasing and pushing the timer button, the unit could be operated as long as the viewer wished. Although these units were extremely popular with customers, radiation doses were high. By the late 1950s, general recognition of the risk of damage to the growing ends of bone and the possible induction of leukemia from the substantial radiation exposure led to the disappearance of the shoe-fitting fluoroscope.

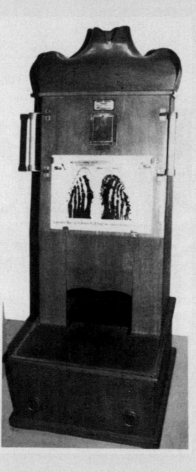

Figure 2-11. Shoe fluoroscope.

that the radiologist could view them in a separate room and eliminate the risk of radiation exposure. Over the next half century, further improvements in screens and image intensifiers, as well as the use of flat-panel detectors, have substantially increased image quality while minimizing the radiation dose to the patient.

What Does the Equipment Look Like?

The fluoroscopic screen and the image intensifier are housed in a metal box that slides over the table so that it can be positioned over the part of the body being examined (Fig. 2-12). The radiologist or technologist uses a foot switch to activate the x-ray source.

What Will You Feel?

The fluoroscopic process itself is simply a different way of producing and recording x-ray images. Therefore, you will not feel anything. Any sensations that you will experience will be related to the examination of which fluoroscopy is a part (such as a barium edema or cardiac catheterization).

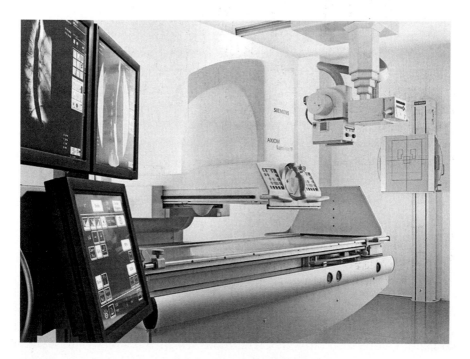

Figure 2-12. Modern fluoroscopy machine. The images are visible on the monitors at the far left.

Advantages and Disadvantages of Fluoroscopy

Advantages

- Real-time imaging
- Ability to reposition the x-ray field instantly during an examination

Disadvantages
- Less detail than ordinary radiographic images

Risks of the Procedure

Examinations using fluoroscopy take much longer to perform than ordinary radiographic studies. Some may take 30 minutes or more compared with an exposure of less than 1 second for a chest or bone radiograph. Consequently, the exposure rate must be kept at a very low level, typically 100–200 times less that used for plain radiographs. This means that the visible fluoroscopic image is created by far fewer x-ray photons, producing a grainy picture with substantially less detail.

The radiologist and technologist take great care to use the lowest radiation dose for the shortest possible time needed to produce diagnostic images. Remember that in a fluoroscopic study x-rays are produced only when the x-ray source is activated, which may be a relatively small percentage of the overall duration of the examination.

Because the developing fetus is especially sensitive to radiation, always tell the technologist if you are or may be pregnant.

Barium Swallow

What Is a Barium Swallow?

Also known as an *esophagram*, a barium swallow is a radiographic study that examines the pharynx (throat) and esophagus, the tube that propels food from the mouth to the stomach. It may be performed separately or as part of an upper GI series (see below), which evaluates the esophagus, stomach, and duodenum. There are two basic types of barium swallow. In a single-contrast study, the esophagus is filled with a milkshake-like suspension of barium—a white, chalky powder that outlines the esophagus so that it can be seen on x-rays. The more sensitive double-contrast study uses a combination of barium and air to coat the lining of the esophagus.

This makes it easier for the radiologist to diagnose small polyps, cancer, and inflammatory disease that may be causing your symptoms.

(For the modified barium swallow, or video esophagram, see the next section.)

A common alternative to the barium swallow is endoscopy, in which a thin, flexible tube (endoscope) is inserted through the mouth and guided down the throat and esophagus to look at the inner lining of these structures.

Why Am I Having this Test?

A barium swallow is performed to diagnose problems affecting the structure or function of the pharynx and esophagus. It may discover the cause of such symptoms as difficulty swallowing (dysphagia), painful swallowing (odynophagia), and heartburn (from reflux of acid contents of the stomach that irritates the inner lining of the esophagus), as well as repeated episodes of pneumonia related to improper functioning of the muscles in the esophageal wall. Your physician may order a barium swallow if your clinical symptoms suggest:

- Structural esophageal abnormalities such as narrowing (stricture) and outpouchings (diverticula) and motility disorders (Fig. 2-13)
- Cancer of the pharynx or esophagus (Fig 2-14)
- Hiatal hernia with gastroesophageal reflux and esophageal ulcers
- Esophageal varices (enlarged veins that may bleed)
- Achalasia (failure of relaxation of the muscle at the end of the esophagus so that food cannot pass easily into the stomach)

What Should You Tell Your Doctor?

Before going for a barium swallow, make certain to tell your doctor if you:

- Are or suspect that you may be pregnant
- Are allergic to barium or any medicine
- Are allergic to any ingredients of the artificial chocolate, berries, or citrus fruit used to flavor the barium mixture

Why Was the Barium Swallow Developed and How Does It Work?

The pharynx and esophagus cannot usually be seen on plain radiographs. The demonstration of abnormalities within these structures requires sharp detail of their inner walls, which can only be produced by barium or a combination of barium and air.

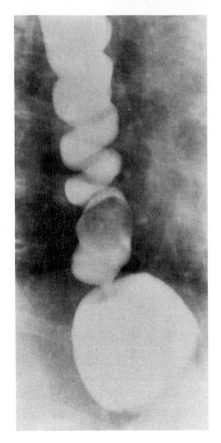

Figure 2-13. Diffuse esophageal spasm.

How Do I Prepare for a Barium Swallow?

You will be asked not to eat or drink anything after midnight the night before the examination. You also should not chew gum or smoke during that time. You may take needed medicine with a small sip of water. If you are a diabetic and take insulin or another medicine for this condition, check with your doctor to determine if the dosage will have to be adjusted while you are not eating.

What Does the Equipment Look Like?

The barium swallow is performed with standard x-ray equipment that includes a fluoroscope. This enables the radiologist or technologist to follow the barium as it is being swallowed and to position you during the procedure so that images can be obtained with minimal obscuration by overlapping structures.

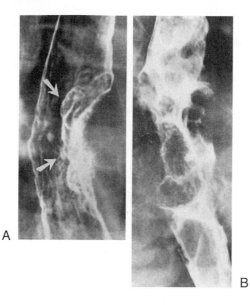

A

B

Figure 2-14. Carcinoma of the esophagus. (A) Localized polpyoid mass with ulcerations (arrow). (B) Bulky irregular filling defect with destruction of mucosal folds.

How Is the Test Performed?

You will be asked to remove any clothing covering your chest and upper abdomen and will be given a lightweight gown to wear. The test usually begins with you standing against the x-ray table, which has been raised to an upright position. As you drink the barium, the radiologist or technologist will observe what is happening using an x-ray fluoroscope, a device that projects the radiographic images like a movie onto a monitor that is similar to a television screen. As the barium (and air) passes through your esophagus, you will be asked to turn into various positions and the examination table will be raised and lowered. (Make sure to tell the person performing the examination if you ever feel uncomfortable or are unable to assume different positions.) When the various sections of the esophagus are adequately coated with barium (and air), the radiologist or technologist will obtain a series of fluoroscopic x-ray images (*spot films*) from various angles. As these pictures are being made, you will be asked to hold still and stop breathing for a few seconds to prevent blurring of the images.

A double-contrast examination of the esophagus may require you to swallow some gas-producing powder followed by a small amount of water. The gas dilates the esophagus and permits the barium to thinly coat the esophageal wall, revealing any erosions, polyps, and even small cancers.

A video may be taken of you swallowing barium if there is a question about the functioning of the esophageal muscles. If there is concern about an area of narrowing that is obstructing the normal passage of food down your esophagus, you may be asked to swallow a small piece of barium-soaked bread or a barium tablet to see whether it gets stuck.

After the fluoroscopic portion of the examination is finished, you may be placed in different positions and given more barium to drink while the technologist takes a routine series of chest radiographs (*overhead views*) with you in different positions. When the examination is complete, you will be asked to wait for a few minutes until the radiologist determines that all the necessary images have been obtained and are technically acceptable.

If there is concern that there may be an esophageal perforation, instead of barium you will be given a nonionic, iodine-containing, water-soluble contrast material, since this is quickly absorbed from adjacent tissue and causes no complications. This material is safe even if it enters your respiratory tubes and is aspirated into your lungs.

A barium swallow usually takes 30 minutes or less. After the test, you may resume your regular diet unless otherwise instructed. If the barium stays in your intestine, it can harden and cause constipation or even a blockage. Therefore, it is important to drink plenty of liquids to help flush it out of your body. Your doctor may suggest that you take a mild over-the-counter laxative.

What Will You Feel?

Some patients find the thick consistency of the barium unpleasant and difficult to swallow. Another common complaint is the chalky taste of the barium, though in many radiology departments this is camouflaged by adding a sweet flavor such as chocolate or strawberry. Lying on the hard examination table and having it tilted into various positions may be uncomfortable. As the fluoroscope is moved into various positions and spot films are exposed, you may hear mechanical noises related to the radiographic equipment.

For a few days after the procedure, barium may make your bowel movements look white or gray. Notify your physician if you have difficulty having bowel movements or are unable to have any for 2 days after the test.

What Are the Advantages and Disadvantages of a Barium Swallow Compared with Endoscopy?

Advantages

- Extremely safe and noninvasive
- No need for sedation

- Better for assessing the swallowing function, muscular abnormalities, and gastroesophageal reflux associated with a hiatal hernia

Disadvantages

- Less sensitive than endoscopy for demonstrating small areas of ulceration or irritation of the lining of the esophagus (esophagitis) and small tumors
- If an abnormality is found during a barium swallow, it can only be removed or biopsied on endoscopy

Risks of the Procedure

Although a barium swallow is generally a safe procedure, the following rare complications can occur:

- Constipation or fecal impaction if the barium is not completely eliminated from the body; therefore, a person with a known gastrointestinal obstruction should not have a barium swallow
- Leakage of barium through a perforation of the esophagus into the tissues of the neck or chest
- Aspiration of barium into the lungs if the person's ability to swallow is greatly impaired

Modified Barium Swallow (Video Esophagram)

This imaging procedure is most commonly performed by a radiologist and a speech therapist if repeated episodes of pneumonia suggest swallowing dysfunction and aspiration of material from the esophagus into the respiratory tract (Fig. 2-15). To closely examine the motion of various structures in the mouth and throat during swallowing, which occurs very rapidly (within about 1–2 seconds), videotapes with a low radiation dose are made in front and side views and analyzed later in slow motion.

Swallowing differs depending on the consistency of the food. Therefore, you will be asked to eat a variety of food types, including thin liquid barium, a thicker mixture with the consistency of pudding, and a solid cracker or cookie that requires chewing and manipulation in the mouth before swallowing. If you have experienced problems with specific types of food, these or similar products can be used to better evaluate your symptoms.

If a swallowing abnormality is identified, the speech therapist may suggest an appropriate treatment strategy to make eating and drinking safer and more efficient. For example, you may be asked to change the position of your head or body before swallowing. At times, merely changing the consistency of the food will allow you to eat safely and prevent aspiration.

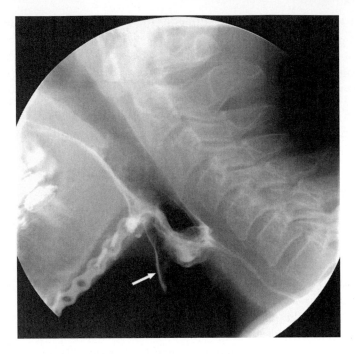

Figure 2-15. Video esophagram. Aspiration of barium from the esophagus into the respiratory tract (arrow) in a patient who had sustained serious facial injuries.

Once a swallowing problem has been identified and therapy begun, a follow-up video esophagram can assess improvement and suggest further modifications of the treatment plan.

Upper GI Series

What Is an Upper GI Series?

An upper GI series is a radiographic examination that produces x-ray images of the upper GI tract, including the esophagus, stomach, duodenum, and first part of the small intestine. There are two basic types of upper GI series. In a single-contrast study, these structures are filled with a suspension of barium. that can be seen on x-rays. The more sensitive double-contrast study uses a combination of barium and air to coat the inside lining of the esophagus, stomach, and duodenum. This makes it easier for the radiologist to diagnose ulcers, tumors, and hernias that may be causing your symptoms.

A common alternative to the upper GI series is endoscopy, in which a thin, flexible tube (endoscope) is inserted through the mouth and guided down the upper GI tract to look at the inner lining of the esophagus, stomach, duodenum, and upper small intestine. In many cases, endoscopy has replaced the upper GI series. In some centers, the upper GI series is now performed primarily to demonstrate complications of weight-reduction (bariatric) surgery, such as excessive narrowing or obstruction of the stomach and perforation through its wall (Fig. 2-16).

Why Am I Having this Test?

An upper GI series is most often performed to discover the cause of such symptoms as difficulty swallowing, vomiting, heartburn, and abdominal pain. Your physician may order an upper GI series if your clinical symptoms suggest:

- Hiatal hernia (causing reflux of acid stomach contents that irritates the inner lining of the esophagus)
- Peptic ulcer
- Tumor
- Obstruction

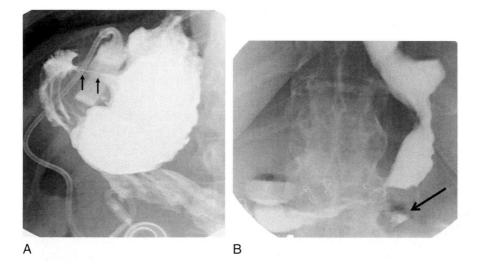

A   B

Figure 2-16. Complications of bariatric surgery. (A) Slipped gastric band causing obstruction (arrow). (B) Leak of contrast material from the stomach (arrow), which was seen fluoroscopically but could not be detected on CT.

What Should You Tell Your Doctor?

Before going for an upper GI series, make certain to tell your doctor if you:

- Are or suspect that you may be pregnant
- Are allergic to barium or any medicine
- Are allergic to any ingredients of the artificial chocolate, berries, or citrus fruit used to flavor the barium mixture

Why Was the Upper GI series Developed and How Does It Work?

Air can be seen within portions of the esophagus, stomach, duodenum, and upper small bowel on plain radiographs of the chest and abdomen. However, the demonstration of abnormalities within these structures requires sharp detail of their inner walls, which can only be produced by coating them with barium or a combination of barium and air.

Historical vignette

In 1910, two Austrian researchers set out to find a GI contrast agent that would be nontoxic, inexpensive, easy to make, and still produce pictures rich in contrast. They settled on pure barium sulfate, which they administered in the form of a chocolate drink.

How Do I Prepare for an Upper GI Series?

To ensure the best possible image, your stomach must be empty. Therefore, you will be asked not to eat or drink anything after midnight the night before your examination. You also should not chew gum or smoke during that time. You may take needed medicine with a small sip of water. If you are a diabetic and take insulin or another medicine for this condition, check with your doctor to see if the dosage will have to be adjusted while you are not eating. If your test is scheduled for the afternoon, you may have a light breakfast (such as dry toast and coffee or tea) before 7 A.M., but do not have anything to eat or drink after that time.

What Does the Equipment Look Like?

The barium enema is performed on standard x-ray equipment that includes a fluoroscope. This enables the radiologist or technologist to follow the barium as it is being swallowed and to position you during the procedure so that images can be obtained with minimal obscuration by overlapping structures.

How Is the Test Performed?

You will be asked to remove any clothing covering your upper abdomen and will be given a lightweight gown to wear. After you lie down on the x-ray table, an initial *scout* view will be taken before you drink any barium. For a double-contrast upper GI series, before drinking the barium you will be asked to swallow some granules that fizz like Alka-Seltzer to increase the air (gas) within your stomach. You may feel the need to belch but try not to do so, since an adequate amount of air is necessary to achieve high-quality images with excellent detail.

As you drink the barium, the radiologist or technologist will observe what is happening using an x-ray fluoroscope, a device that projects the radiographic images like a movie onto a monitor that is similar to a television screen. As the barium and air pass through your esophagus, stomach, and duodenum, you will be asked to turn into various positions and the examination table will be raised and lowered. (Make sure to tell the person performing the examination if you ever feel uncomfortable or are unable to assume different positions.) When the various sections of the upper GI tract are adequately coated with barium and air, the radiologist or technologist will expose a series of spot films from various angles. As these pictures are being made, you will be asked to hold still and stop breathing for a few seconds to prevent blurring of the images. At times, the person performing the examination may press gently on your abdomen with a hand or plastic paddle to separate overlapping portions of the upper GI tract to get the best possible pictures. After the fluoroscopic portion of the examination is finished, in some facilities the technologist will take a standard series of overhead views. When the examination is complete, you will be asked to wait for a few minutes until the radiologist determines that all the necessary images have been obtained and are technically acceptable.

The entire upper GI series usually takes about 30–45 minutes. After the test, you may resume your regular diet unless otherwise instructed. If the barium stays in your intestine, it can harden and cause constipation or even a blockage. Therefore it is important to drink plenty of liquids to help flush it out of your body. Your doctor may suggest that you take a mild over-the-counter laxative.

What Will You Feel?

Some patients find the thick consistency of the barium unpleasant and difficult to swallow. Another common complaint is the chalky taste of the barium, though in many radiology departments this is camouflaged by adding a sweet flavor such as chocolate or strawberry. Lying on the hard examination table and having it tilted into various positions may be uncomfortable, as may having pressure applied to your abdomen. If you are having a double-contrast study, the extra air may make you feel bloated. As the fluoroscope is moved into various positions and the spot films are exposed, you may hear mechanical noises related to the radiographic equipment.

For a few days after the procedure, barium may make your bowel movements look white or gray. Notify your physician if you have difficulty with bowel movements or are unable to have any for 2 days after the test.

What Are the Advantages and Disadvantages of an Upper GI Series Compared with Endoscopy?

Advantages

- Extremely safe and noninvasive
- No need for sedation

Disadvantages

- Less sensitive than endoscopy for demonstrating small areas of ulceration or irritation of the lining of the esophagus (esophagitis) and stomach (gastritis), as well as small tumors
- If an abnormality is found during an upper GI series, it can only be removed or biopsied on endoscopy

Risks of the Procedure

Although an upper GI series is generally a safe procedure, the following rare complications can occur:

- Constipation or fecal impaction if the barium is not completely eliminated from the body; therefore, a person with a known GI obstruction should not have an upper GI series
- Leakage of barium into the abdomen through a perforated ulcer

Small Bowel Series

What Is a Small Bowel Series?

A small bowel series (or small bowel follow-through) is a radiographic examination that produces x-ray images of the jejunum and ileum, the two major portions of the small intestine. It assesses the area beyond that evaluated by an upper GI series. There are two basic types of small bowel series. The first is a traditional single-contrast study, which is usually performed after an upper GI series. The patient is given several additional cups of barium to fill the entire small bowel. However, the length and location of the small intestine lead to overlapping of bowel loops that often produces a confusing picture. A more sensitive test, but one that is more invasive and uncomfortable, is *enteroclysis*. A Greek word that literally means "washing out of the intestine," enteroclysis is a dedicated study that focuses only on the small bowel. In this double-contrast procedure, a tube introduced through the nose is positioned in the small bowel. Both barium and methylcellulose (or air) are injected through the tube to distend the small bowel and coat the inside lining of the jejunum and ileum. The sharp detail produced by enteroclysis makes it easier for the radiologist to detect abnormalities that may be causing your symptoms.

A newer approach is to combine enteroclysis and CT (or MRI). This is reported to be the best technique now available to image the small bowel.

Why Am I Having this Test?

A small bowel series is primarily performed to evaluate and diagnose:

- Malabsorption (diarrhea, cramping, frequent bulky stools, bloating, flatulence [gas], abdominal distention, and nutritional deficiencies)
- Inflammatory disease of the small bowel (especially Crohn's disease) (Fig. 2-17)
- Small bowel obstruction
- GI bleeding
- Tumors

What Should You Tell Your Doctor?

Before going for a small bowel series, make certain to tell your doctor if you:

- Are or suspect that you may be pregnant
- Are allergic to barium or any medicine
- Are allergic to any ingredients of the artificial chocolate, berries, or citrus fruit used to flavor the barium mixture

Why Was the Small Bowel Series Developed and How Does It Work?

Air can be seen within portions of the jejunum and ileum on plain radiographs of the abdomen. However, the demonstration of abnormalities within these structures requires sharp detail of their inner walls, which can only be

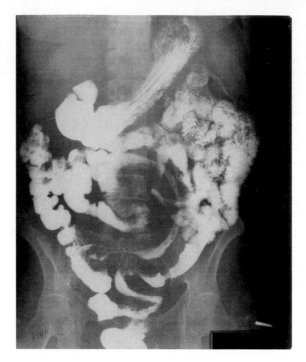

Figure 2-17. Crohn's disease. Single-contrast small bowel series shows a characteristic pattern of multiple areas of severe narrowing (string sign) separated by normal segments (skip lesions).

produced by coating them with barium or a combination of barium and air (or methylcellulose).

How Do I Prepare for a Small Bowel Series?

The preparation for a small bowel series is the same as that for an upper GI series. To ensure the best possible images of the small bowel, you will be asked not to eat or drink anything after midnight the night before the examination. You also should not chew gum or smoke during that time. You may take needed medicine with a small sip of water. If you are a diabetic and take insulin or another medicine for this condition, check with your doctor to determine if the dosage will have to be adjusted while you are not eating.

What Does the Equipment Look Like?

The small bowel series is performed on standard x-ray equipment that includes a fluoroscope. This enables the radiologist or technologist to follow the barium (and methylcellulose or air) as it is being swallowed and to position you during the procedure so that images can be obtained with minimal overlap of bowel loops. In an enteroclysis study, the tube is positioned in the small bowel using the fluoroscope.

How Is the Test Performed?

If a small bowel study is performed in combination with an upper GI series, see the description in that section (p. 44). After the upper GI series is completed, you will be given several more cups of barium to drink. Radiographs will be taken every 15–30 minutes until there has been adequate filling of the entire small bowel. The radiologist may then fluoroscope the end of your small bowel (terminal ileum), which is often involved with inflammatory diseases such as Crohn's disease, pressing gently on your abdomen with a hand or plastic paddle to separate overlapping loops. Then the technologist will take a standard series of overhead views. When the examination is complete, you will be asked to wait for a few minutes until the radiologist determines that all the necessary images have been obtained and are technically acceptable.

For an enteroclysis examination, your throat will be sprayed with a local anesthetic. After asking whether it is easier for you to breathe through one nostril, the technologist will lubricate it with a small amount of Xylocaine jelly or a similar product. Then the radiologist will insert a small-diameter rubber tube through your nose. You may either be sitting or lying down for the initial placement of the catheter, depending on your comfort and the preference of the radiologist. The radiologist will then push the tube through the stomach and into your small intestine, frequently checking its position under the fluoroscope. When the tube is in the proper place, it will be taped to your nose. The tubing is then connected to a machine, which will first administer the barium and then the methylcellulose or air. As the barium flows in, your abdomen may feel bloated. This bloating can often be relieved by taking slow, deep breaths through your mouth. As the barium and methylcellulose (or air) proceed through your small bowel, you may be asked to roll into various positions while the radiologist takes a series of spot films. Then the technologist will take a standard series of overhead views. When the examination is complete, the tube is removed. You will be asked to wait for a few minutes until the radiologist determines that all the necessary images have been obtained and are technically acceptable.

An enteroclysis examination usually takes about 30–45 minutes. Depending on how fast the barium moves through the intestine, a small bowel series may take 1–2 hours or more. After the test, you may resume your regular diet unless otherwise instructed. If the barium stays in your intestine, it can harden and cause constipation or even a blockage. Therefore, it is important to drink plenty of liquids to help flush it out of your body. Your doctor may suggest that you take a mild over-the-counter laxative.

For a few days after the procedure, barium may make your bowel movements look white or gray. Notify your physician if you have difficulty having bowel movements or are unable to have any for 2 days after the test.

CT Enterography and Enteroclysis

These newer studies are performed the same way as the procedures described above, except that the images are obtained by CT rather than plain radiographs. Advantages include the ability to examine bowel loops without superimposition and to evaluate the entire thickness of the bowel wall and the surrounding mesentery and peritoneal fat. These CT procedures are especially valuable for determining the extent and severity of inflammatory bowel disease, primarily Crohn's disease (Fig. 2-18). However, they do not demonstrate the inner lining of the small bowel in as much detail as a small bowel series or enteroclysis.

What Will You Feel?

Some patients find the thick consistency of the barium unpleasant and difficult to swallow. Another common complaint is the chalky taste of the barium, though in many radiology departments this is camouflaged by adding a sweet

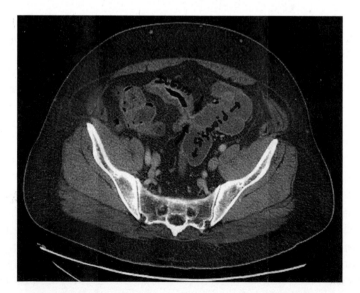

Figure 2-18. CT enteroclysis. In this patient with Crohn's disease, CT of the pelvis demonstrates a fistula between the thick-walled ileum and sigmoid colon.

flavor such as chocolate or strawberry. Lying on the hard examination table, having it tilted into various positions, and having pressure applied to your abdomen may be uncomfortable for some patients. If you are having a double-contrast study, the extra air may make you feel bloated. As the fluoroscope is moved into various positions and the spot films are exposed, you may hear mechanical noises related to the radiographic equipment.

If you have an enteroclysis, passing the tube can be quite uncomfortable, even with the use of anesthetic spray and Xylocaine jelly.

What Are the Relative Advantages of Small Bowel Series and Enteroclysis?

Small Bowel Series

- Noninvasive and painless (no tube is inserted)
- Widely available
- Lower radiation dose

Enteroclysis

- Faster (barium is injected directly into the small bowel, rather than having to wait for the normal movements of the GI tract to get it there)
- Increased distention of the small bowel and sharper detail of the inner lining of the jejunum and ileum produce far superior images that make it easier to detect and characterize abnormalities
- Ability to display all the dilated, contrast-filled loops of small bowel simultaneously at the end of the examination (only segments of the small bowel are visualized at a given time in a small bowel series)

Risks of the Procedure

Although the small bowel series and enteroclysis are generally safe procedures, a rare complication is constipation or fecal impaction (if the barium is not completely eliminated from the body).

Barium Enema

What Is a Barium Enema?

A barium enema, also known as a *lower GI series*, is a radiographic examination that produces x-ray images of the large intestine (colon and rectum). There are two basic types of barium enema examinations. In a single-contrast study, the large intestine is filled with a liquid suspension of barium—a white, chalky powder that outlines the bowel so that it can be seen on x-rays. This is the faster and more comfortable procedure, but it can only demonstrate large abnormalities within the colon. A more sensitive study is the double-contrast (*air-contrast*) enema, in which barium is allowed to fill much of the colon and then drain out, leaving only a thin layer coating the wall. The colon is then filled with air, giving the radiologist a detailed view of the inner surface of the colon. This makes it easier to diagnose small polyps, cancer, and inflammatory disease of the colon and rectum that may be causing your symptoms.

A common alternative to the barium enema is colonoscopy, in which a long, lighted, flexible tube (colonoscope) is inserted through the rectum to view the inside of the colon.

Anatomy of the Colon

The colon is the first 6 feet of the large intestine, which connects with the rectum and then the anus, where waste material passes out of the body. A major role of the colon is to absorb water to form a semisolid stool. The colon is divided into four sections:

- Ascending colon—extends upward on the right side of the abdomen
- Transverse colon—extends across the body from the ascending colon to the left side
- Descending colon—extends from the transverse colon downward on the left side of the abdomen
- Sigmoid colon—named for its S shape, it connects the descending colon and the rectum

Why Am I Having this Test?

A barium enema is primarily performed primarily to detect polyps and cancer in the colon (Fig. 2-19). This may be done as a screening procedure or if you have symptoms such as a change in bowel habits (diarrhea or constipation), blood in the stools, or unexplained weight loss. Your physician may also order a barium enema if your clinical symptoms suggest:

- Inflammatory bowel disease (ulcerative colitis, Crohn's disease)
- Diverticulosis (dilated sacs in the wall of the large intestine) or diverticulitis (inflammation of diverticula, causing narrowed areas in the colon)
- Obstruction of the colon

If your physician suspects that you might have an acute bowel perforation, diverticulitis, or toxic megacolon (a dilated, thin-walled colon, most

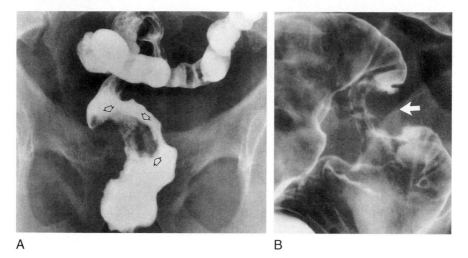

A   B

Figure 2-19. Colorectal cancer. (A) Single-contrast barium enema shows a bulky tumor mass (arrows) that could be felt on rectal examination. (B) Double-contrast study in another patient shows an area of severe narrowing in the sigmoid colon. This malignant "apple-core" lesion is relatively short and has sharply defined margins.

commonly due to ulcerative colitis) but that you require a contrast enema, the radiologist will suggest the use of a water-soluble material instead of barium to decrease the risk of perforation and the extent of complications if a perforation occurs.

What Should You Tell Your Doctor?

Before going for a barium enema, make certain to tell your doctor if you:

- Are or suspect that you may be pregnant
- Are allergic to latex, since products containing latex are commonly used to administer the barium
- Know that you are allergic to barium
- Have had a recent upper GI series or a barium swallow, because residual barium in the colon may cause a confusing appearance. If you need both a barium enema and either an upper GI series or a barium swallow, the barium enema should always be performed first, since it may take several days for swallowed barium to pass through the intestine.

Why Was the Barium Enema Developed and How Does It Work?

Air can be seen within portions of the colon on plain radiographs of the abdomen. However, the demonstration of abnormalities within the colon requires sharp detail of its inner wall, which can only be produced by barium or a combination of barium and air. On single-contrast examinations, polyps in the colon appear as black *filling defects* within the white barium. On double-contrast studies, they appear as masses that are coated by barium and either lie flat along the wall of the colon or are attached to it by a stalk of variable length.

How Do I Prepare for a Barium Enema?

The key to a successful barium enema is a clean colon. Even a small amount of retained stool can reduce the accuracy of the test. Each radiology department has its own special bowel preparation procedure (*prep*) for you to follow before a barium enema. While specific details may vary, this bowel prep usually includes a laxative (a medicine that loosens stool and increases bowel movements) and a suppository (to cleanse the rectum of any remaining fecal material). Some common preparations are the Fleet Prep Kit 1 (phospho-soda and Bisacodyl) and NuLytely or Go-Lytely (polyethylene glycol electrolyte solutions).

You may be asked to consume a low-residue diet for 3 days before the procedure, avoiding fruits, salad, cereal, bran, seeds, and nuts. (Many radiology departments and facilities will give you a detailed list of what you can and cannot eat during this period.) You will probably be asked to have a clear liquid diet for 1–2 days before the barium enema and have nothing to eat or drink for several hours before your appointment. You may take needed medicine with a small sip of water. If you are diabetic and take insulin or another medication for diabetes, check with your doctor to determine if the dosage will have to be adjusted while you are not eating.

What Does the Equipment Look Like?

The barium enema is performed on standard x-ray equipment that includes a fluoroscope. This enables the radiologist or technologist to follow the barium as it is being swallowed and to position you during the procedure so that images can be obtained with minimal overlap of bowel loops.

How Is the Test Performed?

You will be asked to remove any clothing covering the course of the colon and will be given a lightweight gown to wear. After you lie down on the x-ray table, an initial scout view will be taken to make certain that there is no residual barium or excessive retained stool in your colon that would interfere with the study.

As you lie on your side, a well-lubricated enema tube will be inserted gently into your rectum. The barium contrast material is then allowed to flow slowly into your colon. You may feel the need to have a bowel movement, but it is important to resist the urge to allow the barium to leak back out. A small balloon around the enema tip may be inflated to help you hold in the barium. Taking slow, deep breaths and tightening your anal sphincter muscle (as if you were trying to hold back a bowel movement) also may help. If you are very uncomfortable, you may be given an injection of medicine to relieve the cramping.

The radiologist or technologist will observe the barium flowing into your colon using an x-ray fluoroscope monitor that is similar to a television screen. In a double-contrast study, you will be asked to evacuate some of the barium into a bedpan or the toilet. The enema tip will be reinserted and your colon filled with air. During the procedure, you will be asked to turn in different directions and the table may be tilted slightly. This enables the barium to flow throughout your colon and allows the radiologist or technologist to expose a series of spot films with you in various positions. At times, the person performing the examination may press gently on your abdomen with a hand or plastic paddle, either to help move the barium through your colon or to separate overlapping loops of bowel to get the best possible images.

When your colon is filled, the technologist will take a routine series of overhead views of the abdomen. The enema tip is then removed, and you will be given a bedpan or taken to the toilet. After you eliminate as much barium as you can, one or two additional x-ray images (*postevacuation films*) are usually taken to complete the examination. A barium enema usually takes 30–60 minutes, though barium and air will be in your colon only about half of that time.

After the test, you may resume your regular diet unless otherwise instructed. Because the bowel preparation causes you to lose up to 2 quarts of fluid in bowel movements, it is very important that your drink extra fluid on the day that you complete the bowel prep and for 2 days after the examination to help avoid such complications as dizziness and fainting. Because barium may cause constipation or even impaction, drinking large amounts of liquids after the examination helps flush any remaining barium out of your colon. Eating foods high in fiber aids in eliminating the barium from your body; you also may be given a cathartic or laxative.

For a few days after the procedure, barium may make your bowel movements look white or gray. Notify your physician if you:

- Experience severe abdominal pain or distention
- Have difficulty with bowel movements or are unable to have any for 2 days

- Have stools that are smaller in diameter than normal
- Develop rectal bleeding or a fever

What Will You Feel?

A barium enema examination can be uncomfortable. For most people, the long and rigorous bowel prep is the most difficult part of the test. Castor oil and other bowel-cleansing products have an unpleasant taste. The frequent bowel movements can be exhausting, and you should arrange for someone to drive you home after the test. The bowel prep may cause soreness in your anal area, which can be relieved by warm sitz baths or a soothing ointment such as Preparation H.

As the barium flows into your colon, you may feel sensations of fullness and cramping, as well as a strong urge to have a bowel movement. If an air-contrast study is performed, you may experience increased pain and cramping as the gas is introduced into your colon. Taking slow, deep breaths through your mouth can help you relax and decrease the discomfort. It is important to resist the urge to have a bowel movement so that the barium dos not leak out. The radiologist or technologist performing the study can inflate a small balloon around the enema tip to help you hold the barium in; if you are very uncomfortable, you may be given an injection of medicine to relieve the cramping.

What Are the Advantages and Disadvantages of a Barium Enema Compared with Colonoscopy?

Advantages

- Less expensive and fewer risks
- No need for sedation

Disadvantages

- Small polyps are more likely to be missed
- A polyp detected on barium enema can only be removed or biopsied by colonoscopy

Risks of the Procedure

Although barium enema is generally a safe procedure, the following rare complications can occur:

- Constipation or fecal impaction if the barium is not completely eliminated from the body

- Perforation of the colon due to the pressure of barium and air on a portion of the intestinal wall that is weakened by inflammatory bowel disease (such as ulcerative colitis or Crohn's disease)
- Water intoxication due to excess absorption of water into the body from cleansing enemas prior to the procedure

3

ULTRASOUND

Ultrasound

What Is Ultrasound?

Ultrasound, also known as *sonography*, is a noninvasive medical test that uses reflected high-frequency sound waves to produce pictures of organs inside of your body. Ultrasound examinations do not use ionizing radiation (x-rays) and thus are considered safe for pregnant women and children. Captured in real time, ultrasound images show the structure and movement of the body's internal organs, as well as blood flow through arteries and veins.

Why Am I Having this Test?

Your physician has ordered an ultrasound scan because it provides more detailed and precise information about your condition than conventional x-ray examinations. Ultrasound can be used to study any part of the body and search for various conditions:

- Abdomen—tumors, cysts, and abscesses of abdominal organs (liver, pancreas, spleen, kidneys, adrenals); stones in the gallbladder (Fig. 3-1) and kidney; appendicitis; bile duct obstruction causing jaundice; ascites (excess fluid in the abdominal cavity); and to determine the cause of nonspecific abdominal pain
- Pelvis—abnormalities of the uterus, ovaries, and fallopian tubes in women (Figs. 3-2, 3-3) and of the prostate and scrotum (testicles) in men
- Fetus—to monitor the development and detect abnormalities in the unborn child during pregnancy (see "Obstetrical [Fetal] Ultrasound" below)

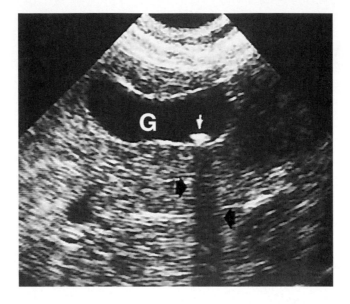

Figure 3-1. Gallstone. The bright echogenic focus (white arrow) seen within an otherwise sonolucent (black) gallbladder (G) represents a large gallstone. Note the characteristic acoustic shadowing immediately below the stone (black arrows).

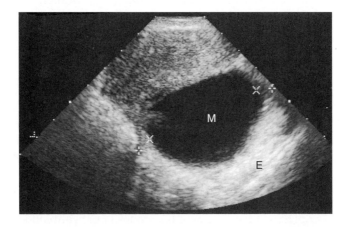

Figure 3-2. Ovarian cyst. Large dark sonolucent mass (M) with enhancement (E) of the back wall within the right ovary.

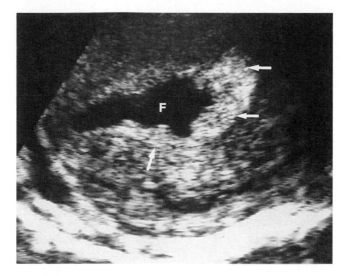

Figure 3-3. Carcinoma of the uterus. There is irregular thickening (arrows) of the inner wall of the uterus (arrows) with a bright echogenic mass (arrowhead) representing the tumor projecting into the fluid-filled endometrial canal (F).

- Breast—to determine whether a mass seen on mammography is cystic (benign) or solid (possibly malignant) (see "Breast Ultrasound," p. 124)
- Neck—tumors, cysts, and abscesses of the thyroid and parathyroid glands; narrowing of the arteries to the brain (Fig. 3-4)
- Legs—narrowing of veins and clots within them (deep venous thrombosis), which can break off and obstruct blood flow to parts of the lungs (pulmonary embolus)
- Blood vessels—aneurysms (abnormally dilated blood vessels, such as the aorta, which supplies blood to the lower part of the body and the legs) and an analysis of the speed and volume of blood flow (see "Doppler Ultrasound" below)
- Heart—chambers and valves of the heart (see "Echocardiography" below); ultrasound also can be used for needle guidance during interventional procedures, such as tissue biopsy, drainage of an abscess, or removal of fluid from the abdominal cavity (paracentesis).

What Should I Tell My Doctor?

Ultrasound has no known risks, and there are no contraindications to the procedure.

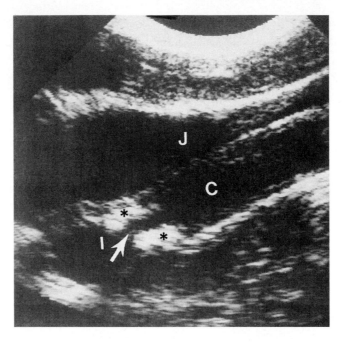

Figure 3-4. Atherosclerotic narrowing of the carotid artery leading to the brain. Ultrasound shows severe narrowing (arrow) of the origin of the internal carotid artery (I) by a densely echogenic (white) arteriosclerotic plaque (asterisks). C, common carotid artery; J, jugular vein.

Why Was Ultrasound Developed and How Does It Work?

Plain radiographs have two important limitations. First, it is impossible to display in a two-dimensional x-ray picture all the information contained in the three-dimensional area being examined. Objects in front of or behind the area of interest are superimposed. This may cause confusion unless lateral (side) or oblique (angled) views are taken. Second, conventional x-rays cannot distinguish among various soft tissues (blood, nerves, muscles, and organs such as the liver, pancreas, and spleen).

Ultrasound imaging uses high-frequency sound waves, which cannot be heard by the human ear, to produce an image of structures inside the body. A transducer (probe) pressed against the skin sends out small pulses of high-frequency sound waves, which reflect off organs, fluids, and tissues within the body and return to a sensitive microphone within the transducer. By measuring these *echo* waves, the ultrasound machine can determine the size and shape of each body structure, how far away it is from the source of the sound, and whether it is solid, filled with fluid, or a combination of both. A computer instantly transforms this material into real-time black-and-white or color moving images on the monitor. A technologist then takes individual still pictures that can be interpreted by the radiologist.

Historical vignette

In 1794, Spallanzani suggested that bats flying in the dark avoid obstacles by being guided by sound (rather than light) produced by the animal that cannot be perceived by the human ear. After the *Titanic* disaster in 1912, high-frequency sound was first used to detect undersea obstacles. This eventually led to the development of sonar (**so**und **na**vigation **a**nd **r**anging) by the United States Navy during World War II. After the war, these techniques began to be applied to diagnostic medical imaging (Fig. 3-5).

How Do I Prepare for an Ultrasound Examination?

You should wear comfortable, loose-fitting clothing for your ultrasound examination. You will be asked to remove all clothing and jewelry in the area to be examined and will be given a lightweight gown to wear during the procedure.

Other preparation depends on the type of ultrasound examination that you will have. For most examinations of the abdomen and pelvis, you will be asked to avoid eating for 8–12 hours before the test to prevent a buildup of gas in the stomach and intestines that could obscure all the structures behind them (since ultrasound waves do not pass through air). For an examination of the liver, gallbladder, spleen, and pancreas, you may be asked to

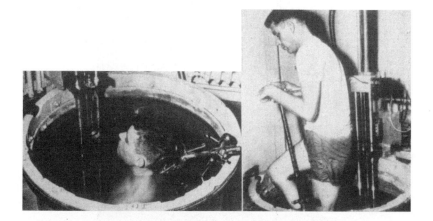

Figure 3-5. Fluid-filled B-29 gun turret scanner (1954). (A) For a transverse cross-section of the neck, the transducer was placed just below the water level. The transducer carriage traveled around the tank on the outside track. (B). The subject stands in the scanner for an examination of the leg.

eat a fat-free meal the evening before the test. If you are scheduled for an ultrasound examination of the kidneys or an obstetrical ultrasound examination, you will be asked to drink several glasses of water or juice about an hour before the examination and avoid urinating so that your bladder will be full (necessary to get a good picture) when the test begins.

What Does the Equipment Look Like?

An ultrasound scanner consists of a computer and a video display screen with a small hand-held transducer that is used to scan the body and blood vessels (Fig. 3-6).

How Is the Test Performed?

In most cases, an ultrasound examination is performed by a technologist (sonographer), who is supervised by a radiologist. You will be asked to lie on your back (or side) on a padded table. A clear, warmed gel is spread on the

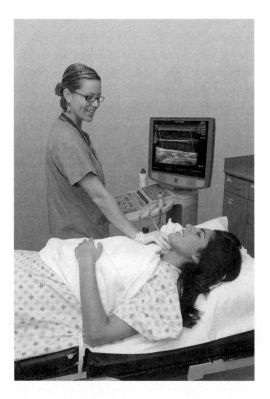

Figure 3-6. Modern ultrasound machine.

area being studied so that the transducer can make secure contact with the body and eliminate air pockets between the transducer and the skin that would degrade the image. The sonographer or radiologist then presses the transducer firmly against the skin and sweeps it back and forth over the area of interest while viewing a picture of the internal organs and blood vessels on a video monitor. You may be asked to change positions for additional scans to be made. For example, for a scan of your kidney, you may be asked to lie on your stomach. At times, you may be asked to take a deep breath and hold it for several seconds (as in an abdominal ultrasound, where this action pushes the liver and spleen lower into the belly so that they are not hidden by the ribs).

For certain ultrasound studies, the transducer is inserted into an opening in your body. For a transesophageal echocardiogram, it is inserted through the mouth into the esophagus to obtain images of the heart. The transducer is inserted into the rectum of a man to study the prostate and into the vagina of a woman to view the uterus and ovaries.

Most ultrasound examinations are completed within 30–60 minutes. When the examination is complete, the gel is wiped off your skin and you can get dressed. You may be asked to wait while the ultrasound images are reviewed by the radiologist to determine whether additional views are necessary. However, the sonographer or radiologist often can review the ultrasound images in real time as they are acquired, allowing you to leave immediately and resume your normal activities.

What Will I Feel?

Most ultrasound examinations are painless and fast. You will not hear or feel the sound waves. The gel spread on your skin may feel cold unless it is first warmed to body temperature. You will feel light pressure from the transducer as it passes over your body. If scanning is performed over an area of tenderness or recent injury, the slight pressure of the transducer may cause some pain.

Ultrasound examinations in which the transducer is inserted into an opening of the body may produce mild discomfort. If a Doppler ultrasound study is performed, you may hear pulse-like sounds that change in pitch as the blood flow is monitored and measured.

What Are the Benefits and Risks of Ultrasound?

Benefits

- Fast, safe, noninvasive (no needles or injections), and usually painless
- Widely available, easy to use, and less expensive than CT or MRI

- No ionizing radiation, making it the imaging modality of choice for pregnant women and their unborn babies (can be repeated as often as necessary)
- Clearly shows soft tissues that do not show up well on x-ray images
- May provide a definitive diagnosis (such as that a mass is a fluid-filled cyst and is definitely benign), thus eliminating the need for additional imaging studies or surgery
- Offers real-time imaging to guide mildly invasive procedures such as needle biopsies and drainages

Risks

- Diagnostic ultrasound has no known harmful effects on humans.

What Are the Limitations of Ultrasound?

- Ultrasound waves do not pass through air and thus are limited in evaluating the bowel or organs that are obscured by overlying gas-filled bowel (CT, MRI, or a barium study is preferred in this setting)
- Contrast material (barium) in the stomach and intestines also prevents passage of the sound waves
- It may be difficult to image obese patients (because tissues decrease the strength of ultrasound waves as they pass deeper into the body)
- Ultrasound waves do not penetrate bones and cannot demonstrate their internal structure (CT or MRI is required)
- Ultrasound is not used to evaluate an open wound, since it is impossible for the transducer to make secure contact with the skin (which is necessary for clear images)

Special Types of Ultrasound

Obstetrical (Fetal) Ultrasound

Ultrasound is performed during pregnancy to produce images of the unborn baby (fetus), the organ that supplies blood and nutrients to it (placenta), and the liquid that surrounds it (amniotic fluid). Unlike x-rays or other types of ionizing radiation that may harm the fetus, ultrasound is the safest way to evaluate the normal development of the unborn baby (size, position) and any possible complications, as well as revealing the sex of the fetus while it is still in the womb.

In many facilities, two routine obstetrical ultrasound scans are obtained. The initial one is an *early risk assessment*, performed at 11–14 weeks of gestation. The second is a *full fetal survey*, performed at approximately 18 weeks. Additional ultrasound examinations may be performed if clinically necessary.

The indications for an obstetrical ultrasound depend on the time during your pregnancy when it is to be performed.

First trimester

- Confirm that the pregnancy is normal and show how the fetus is developing
- Estimate the age of the fetus (gestational age), especially if the date of your last menstrual period is in doubt
- Determine if you are pregnant with more than one fetus (Fig. 3-7)
- Identify any complications (such as ectopic pregnancy or a potential for miscarriage) and early signs of a chromosomal defect, such as Down syndrome
- Check for birth defects affecting the brain or spinal cord (Fig. 3-8)

Second trimester

- Estimate the age, growth, and position of the fetus (and sometimes its gender; Fig. 3-9), as well as whether there are multiple pregnancies (Fig. 3-10)
- Evaluate the appearance and position of the placenta and the amount of amniotic fluid
- Detect major birth defects

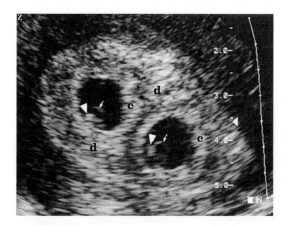

Figure 3-7. Twins. Multiple gestational sacs (dark areas) containing live embryos (arrowhead) at approximately 6.5 weeks.

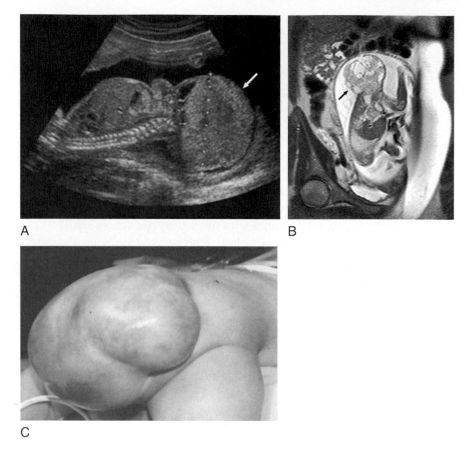

Figure 3-8. Sacrococcygeal teratoma. (A) Ultrasound and (B) MRI show a large mass (arrow) arising adjacent to the base of the spinal canal. (C) Photograph of the newborn infant. Although large, most of these congenital tumors are benign and have a good prognosis.

- Determine the position of the fetus, placenta, and umbilical cord during a diagnostic procedure such as amniocentesis (sampling of the amniotic fluid) or umbilical cord blood sampling

Third trimester

- Evaluate the size and position of the fetus, the appearance of the placenta, and the amount of amniotic fluid
- Make certain that the fetus is alive and moving if there are clinical signs that it is in serious danger

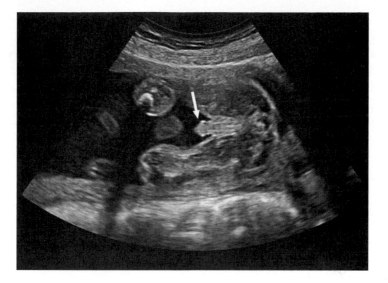

Figure 3-9. Determination of the gender of the fetus. Ultrasound clearly shows the penis (arrow), indicating that the fetus is a male.

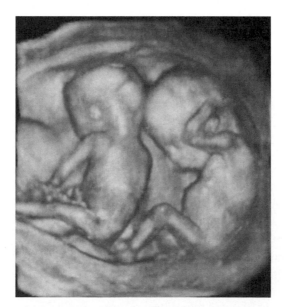

Figure 3-10. Twins. Three-dimensional ultrasound image produced by computer manipulation.

Note: A normal obstetrical ultrasound examination does not guarantee that you will have a normal healthy baby, since birth defects cannot always be detected. If the results of your fetal ultrasound exam are abnormal, your doctor may recommend additional diagnostic tests or procedures to clarify the situation. Although obstetrical ultrasound is considered safe, it should not be performed for a nonmedical reason, such as to identify the sex of the fetus or to obtain a "photograph" of your baby before it is born.

Doppler Ultrasound

Doppler ultrasound is performed to evaluate blood flow in major arteries and veins throughout the body. As examples of its use, Doppler ultrasound can demonstrate:

- An atherosclerotic plaque causing reduction or blockage of blood flow through the carotid arteries in the neck that could cause a stroke
- Blood clots in leg veins (deep vein thrombosis) that could break loose and obstruct blood flow to the lungs (pulmonary embolus)
- Atherosclerotic narrowing of major arteries in the leg with decreased blood flow causing pain with exercise (claudication)
- Whether there is adequate blood flow to a transplanted kidney or liver or increased flow to a hypervascular tumor (Fig. 3-11)

This imaging technique is based on the Doppler effect, a change in the pitch of sound waves arising from a moving object. A common example is the sound of a siren produced by a vehicle (such as a police car or ambulance) as it approaches an observer and then moves away. The frequency of the sound increases as it approaches, is unchanged at the moment it passes by, and decreases as the vehicle moves away. In Doppler ultrasound, the transducer sends out sound waves that bounce back from solid objects such as blood cells. If there is flow of blood within a vessel, there is a change in the pitch of the sound waves that reflect back to the transducer. If there is decreased or no movement of blood cells within a vessel due to venous or arterial narrowing or obstruction, there is no change in the pitch of the sound waves. The computer takes this information and transforms it into a picture that represents the flow of blood through the arteries and veins in the area being examined.

A more complex Doppler machine (color Doppler) converts the reflected sounds into colors that are overlaid on an image and represent the speed and

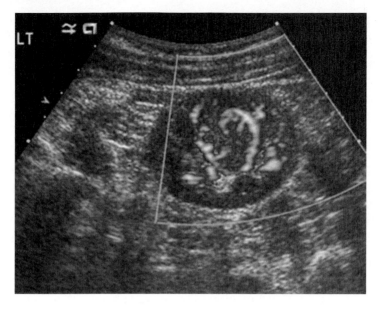

Figure 3-11. Doppler ultrasound. Markedly increased blood flow to a large, hypervascular renal cell carcinoma involving much of the right kidney.

direction of blood flow through arteries and veins. A newer and much more sensitive ultrasound technique is power Doppler, which can evaluate blood flow through the arteries and veins in solid organs and help determine whether a mass is benign or malignant.

Doppler ultrasound is fast, painless, and inexpensive, unlike catheter angiography (see p. 163), which is a complicated, expensive, and somewhat uncomfortable x-rays test that requires the injection of contrast material. However, less-invasive magnetic resonance angiography (see p. 180) and computed tomography angiography (see p. 172) have now replaced conventional angiography for diagnostic purposes.

Echocardiography

Echocardiography is an ultrasound procedure in which sound waves are used to produce a moving picture of the heart. The images are much more detailed than plain x-rays and involve no radiation exposure.

In transthoracic echocardiography (the most common form), the transducer is moved to various locations on the chest or abdominal wall to search for the cause of abnormal heart sounds (murmurs or clicks), an enlarged heart, unexplained chest pain, shortness of breath, or irregular heartbeats. This technique can:

- Measure the size and shape of the chambers of the heart
- Evaluate the thickness and movement of the heart wall
- Assess the working of the heart valves
- Determine how well the heart is performing by calculating the amount of blood it is pumping during each heartbeat (ejection fraction).
- Identify congenital heart defects and the cause of heart failure
- Detect a collection of fluid around the heart (pericardial effusion; Fig. 3-12) or thickening of the fibrous tissue around the heart (pericardium)
- Check the function of the heart after a heart attack
- Determine the function of a new heart valve after surgery

A stress echocardiogram determines whether there is reduced blood flow to the heart muscle (ischemia). This is most commonly related to coronary artery disease. Reduced blood flow is accentuated after some type of stress, usually exercise or ingestion of a medication that makes the heart beat stronger and faster.

A Doppler echocardiogram measures how blood flows through the heart chambers, as well as the pressure and flow across heart valves and within

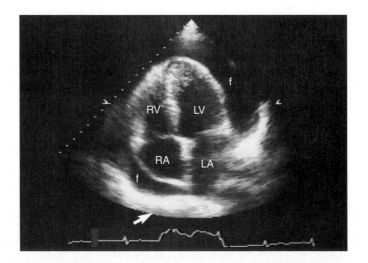

Figure 3-12. Pericardial effusion. Echocardiogram demonstrates an apical four-chamber image of the heart. LA, left atrium; LV, left ventricle; RA, right atrium; RV, right ventricle. The pericardial effusion around the heart (f) produces enhancement of its back wall (arrow).

the major blood vessels entering and exiting the heart. The Doppler measurements may be displayed in black and white or in color.

In a transesophageal echocardiogram, an ultrasound probe is passed down the esophagus rather than moved over the outside of the chest wall. Positioning the probe close to the heart produces a much sharper image, since the sound waves do not have to pass through the lungs and bones of the chest wall. To ease insertion of the transducer into the esophagus, the throat may be numbed with an anesthetic spray, gargle, or lozenge that reduces the gag reflex. In addition to demonstrating abnormalities involving the heart muscle, heart valves, and blood flow, a transesophageal echocardiogram can detect a tear in the wall of the aorta (aortic dissection).

4

COMPUTED TOMOGRAPHY

Computed Tomography

What Is Computed Tomography (CT)?

Computed tomography scanning, also known as *computed axial tomography* (CAT) scanning, is a noninvasive, painless diagnostic test that helps physicians diagnose and treat various medical conditions. It uses sophisticated computer equipment to transform multiple x-ray pictures into *slices* through the body that are displayed on a monitor and can even provide three-dimensional images.

Why Am I Having this Test?

Your physician has ordered a CT scan because it provides more detailed and precise information than plain x-ray examinations for detecting the cause of your symptoms. Computed tomography scans can be used to study any part of the body and search for a broad spectrum of conditions, such as:

- Chest—cancer of the lung (either arising in the lung or spreading to the lung from elsewhere in the body), pulmonary embolism, aortic aneurysm or dissection (Fig. 4-1)
- Abdomen—tumors, cysts, or abscesses of the abdominal organs (liver, pancreas, spleen, kidneys, adrenals; Fig. 4-2); stones in the kidneys, ureters, or bladder; intestinal obstruction and perforation; diverticulitis and appendicitis; bile duct obstruction causing jaundice
- Pelvis—abnormalities of the uterus and ovaries in women and of the prostate and seminal vesicles in men
- Head—stroke (Fig. 4-3), brain injury, tumor, infection, ruptured aneurysm, and other causes of such symptoms as headaches, paralysis, confusion, altered sensation, and vision and hearing problems

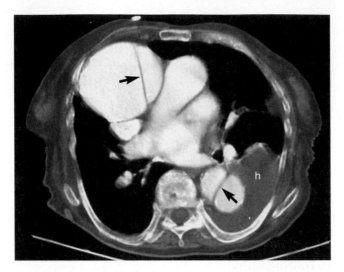

Figure 4-1. Aortic dissection. The ascending aorta (left) is dilated and has a black intimal flap (arrow). The descending aorta (left) has a much larger tear with extensive surrounding hemorrhage (h).

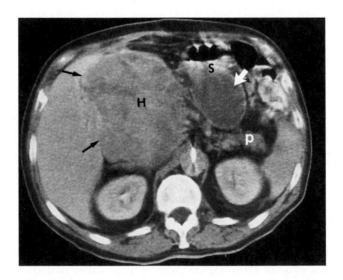

Figure 4-2. Primary cancer of the liver. The huge mass (H) is slightly darker than normal liver. The black arrows point to the junction between the tumor and the normal liver. Incidentally noted is a pancreatic pseudocyst (white arrow) between the stomach (S) and pancreas (p).

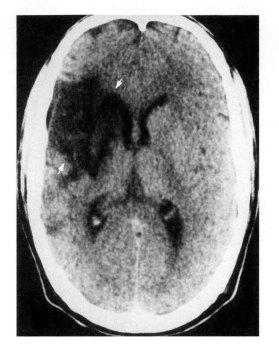

Figure 4-3. Stroke. The low-attenuation (dark) region with a sharply defined border (arrows) represents an old brain infarct in the area supplied by the right middle cerebral artery.

- Spine—herniated disc, spinal stenosis (narrowing of the spinal canal), osteoporosis and compression fractures, spinal tumors and infection
- Bone—detection of subtle fractures that cannot be seen on plain radiographs and evaluation of complex fractures (Fig. 4-4), especially around joints (CT can reconstruct the area of interest in multiple planes; Fig. 4-5)

Computed tomography also can be used to guide a needle during interventional procedures, such as tissue biopsy or drainage of an abscess, and to determine how far a cancer has spread (*staging* the tumor).

What Should I Tell My Doctor?

Before going for a CT scan, make certain to tell your doctor if you:

- Have ever had a reaction to iodinated contrast material from a previous procedure
- Are or might be pregnant or are breast feeding
- Are allergic to foods containing iodine (such as shrimp and other shellfish)

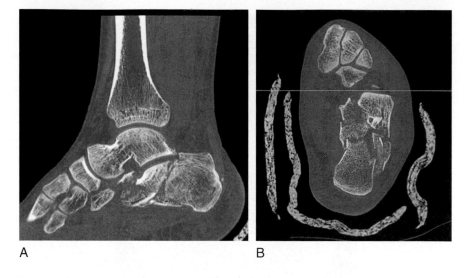

A   B

Figure 4-4. Complex fracture. (A) Lateral and (B) axial views of the foot and ankle show a complex fracture of the calcaneus (heel bone).

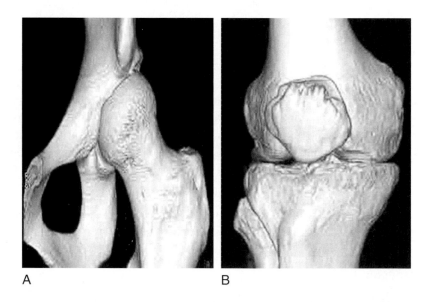

A   B

Figure 4-5. Three-dimensional (3D) CT reconstructions of a normal hip (A) and knee (B).

- Are allergic to any medicine
- Have diabetes or are taking metformin (Glucophage) for diabetes
- Have asthma, kidney, or thyroid problems or multiple myeloma
- Have metallic objects in your body (such as surgical clips or joint replacements) that might obscure the image
- Have recently had an x-ray test using barium (such as a barium enema or an upper GI series), since this dense contrast material may obscure the image and require postponement of the CT study for a few days
- Become nervous when in small spaces (claustrophobia); if so, you may need a sedative to relax (and should arrange for someone to take you home after the procedure)

Why Was CT Developed and How Does It Work?

Plain radiographs have two important limitations. First, it is impossible to display in a two-dimensional x-ray picture all the information contained in the three-dimensional area being examined. Objects in front of or behind the area of interest are superimposed, which may cause confusion unless lateral (side) or oblique (angled) views are taken. Second, conventional x-rays cannot distinguish among various soft tissues (blood, nerves, muscles, and organs such as the liver, pancreas, and spleen) unless contrast material is used.

To overcome these drawbacks, Godfrey Hounsfield developed CT, for which he was awarded the Nobel Prize in Medicine in 1979. Rather than producing an image by using a single detector (film) and a single x-ray source (tube), with CT there are numerous x-ray beams and a set of electronic detectors that rotate about the body and measure the amount of radiation being absorbed at multiple locations as the examination table moves through the scanner. A special computer program processes this huge number of pictures to create two-dimensional sections through the body that are displayed on a monitor. A good way of imagining this process is to think of a loaf of bread being cut into many thin slices, with each CT section representing one thin slice of the body.

Modern CT scanners obtain multiple slices in a single rotation. Known as *multidetector* or *multislice imaging*, continual CT scanning is performed as the patient is moved through a sophisticated array of up to 64 rows of detectors (some 320-row scanners are now available). This permits incredibly fast scanning with substantial reduction of artifacts due to respiratory and cardiac motion. This speed is valuable for all patients, but especially for children, the elderly, and the critically ill. Depending on the diagnostic task, the multiple sections also allow the machine to create three-dimensional images and to format the material in the coronal (frontal-to-back) and sagittal (side-to-side) planes.

CT completely eliminates the superimposition of images of structures outside the area of interest. The inherent high-contrast resolution of CT makes it possible to distinguish between tissues that differ in physical density by less than 1%. Data from a single CT imaging procedure consisting of either multiple contiguous scans or one helical scan can be viewed as images in the axial, coronal, or sagittal planes, depending on the diagnostic task. This is referred to as *multiplanar reformatted imaging*.

Historical vignette

The earliest CT units had a single x-ray source and a detector that slowly turned around the body. Each parallel slice took more than 5 minutes to produce and another 2.5 hours for the computer to generate the final images. Today a single slice through the body requires less than 5 seconds, and almost all CT units take more than one slice at the same time.

How Do I Prepare for a CT Scan?

You should wear comfortable, loose-fitting clothing, though you may have to take off some of your clothes. You will be given a lightweight gown to wear during the procedure. Because metal objects such as eyeglasses, dentures, hairpins, and jewelry can produce artifacts that degrade the image, they may have to be removed, depending on the part of your body being examined. For a CT scan of the abdomen, you may be asked to drink a dilute barium mixture to make it easier for the radiologist to distinguish between the bowel and other adjacent structures.

If you are to receive intravenous contrast material (often popularly known as *dye*), you will be asked to fast (no solids or liquids) for 4–6 hours before the examination. This is necessary to prevent aspiration of stomach contents into the lungs if you have a contrast reaction, which is fortunately uncommon.

Remember that the CT scanner has a weight limit to prevent damage to its internal mechanisms. If you weigh more than 350 pounds, it is possible that you may not be able to have the test performed.

What Does the Equipment Look Like?

A CT scanner consists of three parts, two of which you will actually see. The machine itself looks like a large doughnut, which contains the many x-ray tubes and electronic detectors located opposite each other in a ring (gantry) that rotates around you. You will be placed on a movable examination table, which slides into and out of the center of the machine (Fig. 4-6). The third part of the CT scanner is the sophisticated computer that processes all the imaging information, but it is located in a separate room.

How Is the Test Performed?

You will be asked to lie on the narrow table that slides into the center of the scanner. Most CT scans are taken with you lying on your back, though occasionally it is necessary to lie face down or on your side. If you are to receive intravenous contrast material, it will be injected through a small tube that is usually placed in a small vein of your hand or arm. The number of doses of contrast material and the precise timing vary, depending on the area of the body examined. For a few examinations of the abdomen and pelvis, contrast material is administered through a tube into your bladder or rectum. For some orthopedic studies, contrast material is given through a thin needle placed in a joint.

The first step is for the technologist to take a scout image to test the radiographic technique and to determine the correct starting position for the

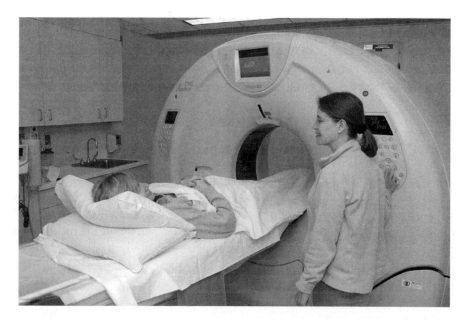

Figure 4-6. CT scanner.

actual CT scan. For this brief part of the procedure, the table moves quickly through the scanner. When the actual CT scan is performed, the table moves more slowly through the machine. To prevent motion that blurs the image, the technician will tell you when to hold your breath and not move. With most modern multidetector scanners, the examination itself is completed within 15 seconds. However, you will be asked to wait for several minutes until the technologist determines that the study is of sufficiently high quality for the radiologist to interpret. Depending on the type of CT scan, the interval between your placement on the table and the time you leave is generally between 10 and 30 minutes.

What Will I Feel?

The x-rays in a CT scan are painless. The main cause of discomfort will probably be the need to lie still on the hard examination table. If the room is too cool, you can ask for a blanket. If you have chronic pain or are claustrophobic, tell the technologist; you may be able to receive medication to ease the pain or let you relax.

When placed on the examination table for the scout film, you may notice special lights designed to make certain that you are in the proper position. During the actual CT scan, there will be a slight metallic sound (buzzing, clicking, whirring) as the gantry revolves around you.

Although you are alone in the CT room during the examination, the technologist will always be able to see you through special leaded glass and answer any questions through a two-way intercom. Parents may be permitted to remain in the examination room with children, though they will be required to wear a lead apron to prevent radiation exposure.

When the CT examination is completed, you can return to your normal activities.

If You Are Given Contrast Material

If you receive intravenous contrast material, you may feel a slight burning sensation in the arm in which it is injected, a metallic taste in the mouth, and a warm flushing of the body. These sensations are normal and usually subside within a few seconds. The most common complication of contrast material is itching and hives, which is relieved with medication. Some patients may feel sick to their stomach. If you become light-headed or have difficulty breathing, notify the technologist immediately, since this may indicate a more severe allergic reaction. In this infrequent occurrence, a radiologist or another physician is always available to provide immediate assistance.

If you are given contrast material to swallow, it may have a mildly unpleasant taste. Contrast given by enema causes a sense of fullness in your abdomen and a feeling that you need to go to the bathroom, but this mild discomfort will soon pass.

After the procedure, you will be asked to drink a large amount of water over the next few hours to clear the contrast material from your body.

What Are the Benefits and Risks of CT Scanning?

Benefits

- Noninvasive and painless
- Extremely fast and ideal for the emergency room setting, as well as for patients who are young, elderly, or critically ill (the entire chest or abdomen can be scanned in less time than it takes to put a patient on the table)
- Offers exquisite anatomic detail
- Distinguishes among various soft tissues (blood, nerves, muscles, various organs), unlike plain radiographs, and shows lungs and bones
- Using computer reconstruction, the data from a single CT imaging procedure can be viewed as images in the axial, coronal, or sagittal planes (multiplanar reformatted imaging) and can even be used to generate beautiful three-dimensional images that can be rotated at various angles
- Compared to MRI, CT is less expensive and less sensitive to patient motion, and can be performed even if you have an implanted metallic medical device
- Offers real-time imaging for mildly invasive procedures such as needle biopsies and drainages
- May provide a definitive diagnosis and eliminate the need for surgical biopsy or exploratory surgery

Risks

- As an x-ray procedure, the multiple slices obtained in a single study have raised questions about the level of radiation exposure. Although there is always a slight chance of developing cancer from radiation, this minuscule theoretical risk is usually far outweighed by the benefits of an accurate diagnosis for a current condition. If you are concerned about this risk, talk to your doctor to confirm that the test is needed and whether there is an alternative study that provides similar information without any radiation exposure.

- Generally not recommend for pregnant women; children should have CT scans only if the diagnosis cannot be made by other studies that do not use x-rays.
- If you have diabetes or are taking the popular anti-diabetes drug metformin (Glucophage), contrast material can cause problems. Your doctor will tell you when you should stop taking metformin before the CT scan and when you can begin to take it again after the test is completed.
- Rare risk of a serious allergic reaction to the contrast material

Special Types of CT

Chest CT

Computed tomography of the chest is often used to further investigate abnormalities detected on plain chest radiographs. This technique is especially valuable for characterizing pulmonary nodules to determine whether they are benign or malignant. In patients with lung cancer, CT can demonstrate the spread of tumor to lymph nodes and the chest wall, as well as monitor the response to treatment. If there is a primary malignancy elsewhere in the body, chest CT is the most accurate method for detecting metastases to the lungs (Fig. 4-7). Following trauma, CT is the best study for showing injury to the chest such as lung contusion or bleeding, damage to the aorta, pneumothorax, and fractures of the ribs and spine. Computed tomography is the ideal imaging test to evaluate patients with emphysema, bronchiectasis, and diffuse interstitial lung disease, as well as diseases of the pleura and chest wall. Biopsies of suspected lung tumors and drainage of abnormal fluid collections in the chest are usually performed under CT guidance.

Abdominal CT

Computed tomography of the abdomen is most commonly used to diagnose the cause of abdominal or pelvic pain and diseases related to the alimentary tract (stomach, small bowel, and colon), urinary tract (kidneys, ureters, bladder), and solid organs such as the liver, spleen, pancreas, and adrenal glands. It is the best modality for demonstrating infectious processes such as appendicitis, diverticulitis, pyelonephritis, and abdominal abscesses, as well as inflammatory conditions such as ulcerative colitis, Crohn's disease, and pancreatitis. Computed tomography has high accuracy in diagnosing

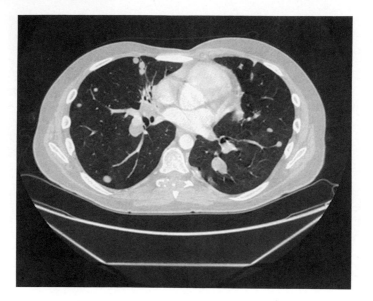

Figure 4-7. Lung metastases. Multiple white nodules of various sizes throughout both lungs.

kidney, ureteral, and bladder stones as well as primary and metastatic malignant tumors involving any of the abdominal organs (Fig. 4-8). In patients with trauma, CT is a rapid and accurate test for identifying injuries to the liver, spleen, and kidneys. Computed tomography is used to guide biopsies and abscess drainages throughout the abdomen and pelvis.

Head CT

Computed tomography of the head is most commonly used to demonstrate acute bleeding following trauma or to diagnose the cause of sudden severe headache in a patient suspected of having a ruptured or a leaking cerebral aneurysm (Fig. 4-9). After injury, head CT is the most accurate technique for detecting fractures of the skull and facial bones as well as acute brain damage. In patients with symptoms of a stroke, CT can demonstrate areas of decreased blood flow and brain infarction. For chronic neurologic conditions, including unexplained seizures and headache, CT generally has been replaced by MRI.

Spine CT

Computed tomography of the spine is the most accurate imaging procedure to determine whether an injury to the back has caused a fracture or other

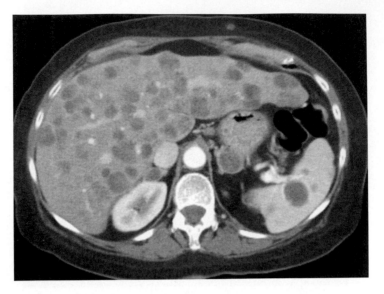

Figure 4-8. Abdominal metastases. Multiple dark rounded areas in the liver, spleen, and left adrenal gland represent diffuse metastases.

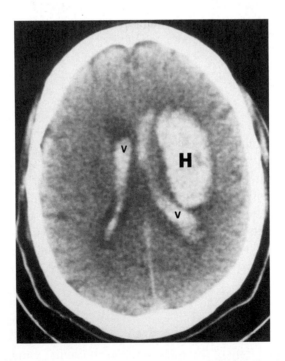

Figure 4-9. Intracerebral hematoma. The large homogeneous high-density area (H) in the brain parenchyma is associated with acute bleeding into the ventricles (v).

damage to the spinal column. Computed tomography can also be used to detect malignant tumors originating in the spinal vertebrae or metastasizing to them. This modality can be used to help diagnose herniated intervertebral disks, spinal stenosis, and other causes of chronic back pain, though in many cases MRI has replaced CT for this purpose.

Whole-body CT Screening

Whole-body CT, which has been advocated as a screening tool for detecting cancer and other diseases in asymptomatic individuals, is a highly controversial concept. Those recommending this study appeal to potential patients by stressing that it is comforting to know that one is disease-free, but if there is evidence of a serious medical condition, it is important to know about it early so that it can be better treated.

The problem is that whole-body CT screening is not simple. The procedure is expensive and could possibly increase the chance of causing cancer from radiation exposure. If a person has no symptoms of illness, there is a high probability that there is nothing seriously wrong and no need for a CT scan to confirm that. In some cases, early detection has little effect on the overall course of the disease. Whole-body CT screening leads to the discovery of numerous findings that will not ultimately affect a patient's health (false positives), but instead will require unnecessary additional follow-up examinations and treatments (including surgery), significant wasted expense, and possible grave complications.

Although whole-body CT screening was popular for several years, most physicians do not recommend these studies unless a person has a specific risk for a certain disease. Major radiology societies have determined that this is not an effective screening method. The need for unnecessary further testing may make the procedure more harmful than beneficial and increases health care costs.

Virtual Colonoscopy

What Is Virtual Colonoscopy?

Virtual colonoscopy, also known as *CT colonography*, is a medical imaging procedure to evaluate the colon (large intestine) from the end of the small bowel to the rectum. Two-dimensional images obtained with CT are transformed by a sophisticated computer into an animated three-dimensional model in which the radiologist views the inside of the large intestine in a way that simulates traveling through the colon.

Why Am I Having this Test?

Your physician has ordered this test to evaluate your colon. The major reason for performing virtual colonoscopy is to screen for polyps, small growths that arise from the inner lining of the large intestine and may become cancerous (Fig. 4-10). The idea is to detect these polyps at an early premalignant stage so that they can be removed before they have a chance to develop into a cancer (Fig. 4-11).

Many physicians agree that everyone older than 50 years of age should be screened for colonic polyps every 7 to 10 years. For those at increased risk, screening is recommended every 5 years and often starts by age 40. Risk factors for developing colon cancer include:

- A personal history of polyps
- A family history of colon cancer
- The presence of blood in the stool

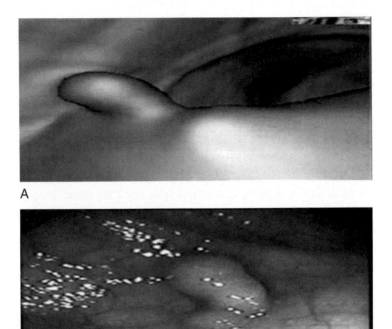

A

B

Figure 4-10. Colonic polyp. (A) CT and (B) optical colonography clearly demonstrate this benign pedunculated polypoid mass.

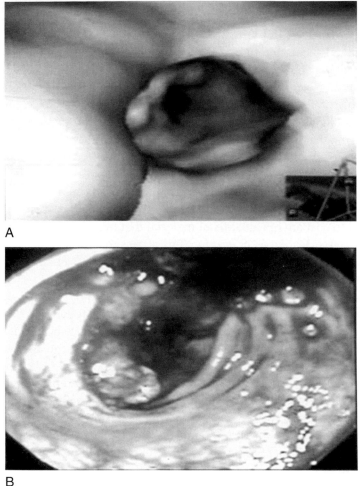

A

B

Figure 4-11. Carcinoma of the colon. (A) CT and (B) optical colonography show this malignant tumor almost occluding the lumen of the colon.

Why Was Virtual Colonoscopy Developed and How Does It Work?

For years, the only type of colonoscopy available used a long, lighted, flexible tube (colonoscope) to view the inside of the colon. However, this technique takes a relatively long time and requires heavy sedation. Also, it may be impossible to see parts of the colon beyond any area that is narrowed due to inflammation or malignancy. Virtual colonoscopy using CT is fast, requires no sedation, and is not limited by narrowing of the colon.

How Do I Prepare for Virtual Colonoscopy?

The key to a successful virtual colonoscopy is a clean colon that is free of any retained fecal material so that the radiologist can clearly detect any polyps that may be present. To accomplish this, your doctor or the radiology department or facility will give you a set of instructions known as a *bowel prep*, which tells you what to do the day or night before the examination. While specific details may vary, this bowel prep usually includes a laxative (a medicine that loosens stool and increases bowel movements) and a suppository (to cleanse the rectum of any remaining fecal material). Some common preparations are the Fleet Prep Kit 1 (phospho-soda and Bisacodyl) and NuLytely or Go-Lytely (polyethylene glycol electrolyte solutions).

As the last step in the preparation process, you may be given a solution designed to coat any residual fecal material that may not have been cleared by the laxative. Called *fecal tagging*, this allows the radiologist viewing the three-dimensional images to effectively ignore any leftover stool that might otherwise mimic a polyp and give a false-positive result.

Before taking a bowel prep, be sure to tell your physician if you have heart, liver, or kidney disease that might make it unsafe. On the day before the examination, you should limit your food intake to clear liquids such as broth, tea, or juice. As soon as the virtual colonoscopy is finished, you may resume your usual diet.

Some radiology departments or facilities use lighter preparations for virtual colonoscopy. These consist of a low-residue diet (such as rice, mashed potatoes, and clear soups) for 3 days. During the last 2 days, barium is mixed into the food. On the radiographic images, this barium coats any polyps but permeates throughout residual fecal material, thus helping the radiologist to distinguish between these often confusing causes of filling defects.

As with all radiology examinations, women should always inform their physician and the CT technologist if there is any possibility that they are pregnant.

How Is the Test Performed?

The technologist will ask you to lie on your back on the CT table. If necessary, straps and pillows may be used to help you maintain the correct position and hold still during the examination. A very small, flexible tube will be passed about 2 inches into your rectum to allow air to be gently pumped into the colon using a hand-held squeeze bulb. Sometimes an electronic pump is used to deliver carbon dioxide gas into the colon. The purpose of the gas is to distend the colon as much as possible to eliminate any folds or wrinkles that might obscure polyps from the radiologist's view.

Next, the table will move through the scanner while a series of two-dimensional cross sections are made along the length of the colon. You will be asked to hold your breath for about 15 seconds before turning over and lying on your side or on your stomach while a second pass is made through the scanner. In some centers, the sequence of positions may be the opposite (facing down first and then up). Once all the images have been taken, the tube is removed. The entire examination is usually completed within 10–15 minutes, and you then can resume your normal activity.

If the radiologist detects an abnormality on your virtual colonoscopy exam, you will probably be asked to undergo a conventional optical colonoscopy, either the same day or at a later time.

What Will I Feel?

Most patients who have virtual colonoscopy report a feeling of fullness when the colon is inflated during the exam, as if they need to pass gas. Less than 5% complain of significant pain. Very infrequently, a muscle-relaxing drug may need to be injected intravenously or subcutaneously to lessen the discomfort. The actual scanning procedure is completely painless.

You will hear a slight buzzing, clicking, or whirring sound as the CT scanner revolves around you during the imaging process. Although you will be alone in the examination room during the CT scan, the technologist is always able to see, hear, and speak with you.

How Does Virtual Colonoscopy Compare to Conventional Optical Colonoscopy?

Advantages

- Minimally invasive test that requires the placement of only a small, thin tube into the rectum to inflate the large intestine, rather than placement of a large colonoscope throughout the entire length of the colon
- Much more comfortable (only a feeling of fullness); consequently, there is no need for sedation and no recovery period, so you can resume your normal activities or go home immediately after the procedure without the help of another person
- Less expensive and much faster
- Can detect polyps and other abnormalities as clearly as conventional optical colonoscopy
- Tolerated much better by the frail and elderly

- Excellent alternative for patients with medical conditions (such as severe breathing difficulties and therapy with blood thinners) that increase the risk of optical colonoscopy
- Substantially lower risk of perforating the colon
- Eliminates two major problems of optical colonoscopy: (1) inability to evaluate the cecum and the right side of the colon adequately in 10% of cases and (2) inability to visualize the entire colon if the bowel is narrowed or obstructed by a large tumor or an inflammatory process
- Can also demonstrate abnormalities outside the colon

Disadvantages

- A purely diagnostic examination that does not allow the radiologist to take tissue samples (biopsy specimens) or remove a polyp during the procedure; therefore, if an abnormality is detected, conventional colonoscopy must also be performed
- Does not consistently detect precancerous polyps smaller than 10 millimeters
- Exposes the patient to radiation
- May be impossible to perform on obese people who are too large to fit into the opening of the CT scanner or are over the weight limit for the moving table
- Many health insurance plans do not pay for virtual colonoscopy as a screening test for colonic polyps, though they may cover the cost if the patient has symptoms related to the colon
- As a new technology, virtual colonoscopy is not as widely available

---

Virtual Bronchoscopy

A similar but less widely used technique is virtual bronchoscopy, which provides detailed, noninvasive images of the airways (trachea and bronchi). This procedure offers information similar to that of conventional bronchoscopy, in which a long, lighted, flexible tube (bronchoscope) is used to view the inside of the airways. However, virtual bronchoscopy is much more comfortable, faster, and less expensive.

5

MAGNETIC RESONANCE IMAGING

Magnetic Resonance Imaging

What Is Magnetic Resonance Imaging (MRI)?

Magnetic resonance imaging is a noninvasive test that uses a powerful magnetic field and pulses of radio wave energy to make detailed pictures of organs and other structures inside the body. In many cases, the unique features of MRI allow this technique to provide different information than plain radiographs, ultrasound, and CT. Magnetic resonance imaging also may show abnormalities that cannot be seen with other imaging methods.

Magnetic resonance imaging uses multiple imaging sequences to characterize various tissues within the body. On T1-weighted images, substances causing high (bright) signal intensity include fat, subacute hemorrhage (Fig. 5-1), highly proteinaceous material (e.g., mucus), and slow-flowing blood. Water, as in cerebrospinal fluid or simple cysts, has relatively low signal intensity and appears dark (Fig. 5-2A). Soft tissue has an intermediate level of signal. On T2-weighted images, water has a high (bright) signal intensity (Fig. 5-2B), whereas muscle and other soft tissues (including fat) tend to have low signal intensity and appear dark. Bone, calcium, and air appear very dark on all imaging sequences.

Magnetic resonance imaging has emerged as the imaging modality of choice for evaluating the central nervous system (brain and spinal cord), musculoskeletal system (including joints and spine), pelvis, retroperitoneum, mediastinum, and large vessels. It is equivalent to contrast-enhanced CT for studying focal liver disease and disorders of the spleen, pancreas, and kidneys. In specific clinical situations, such as most disease processes involving the central nervous system, it is more cost-effective to perform MRI as the initial imaging procedure to achieve a precise diagnosis rather

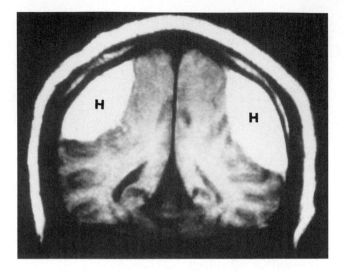

Figure 5-1. Bilateral subdural hematomas. Coronal MR image shows the high signal intensity of these collections of blood on both sides (H).

than obtaining numerous other imaging studies and then having to order an MRI scan anyway. Magnetic resonance imaging has also become the problem-solving modality in fetal imaging, because it can provide much more information than ultrasound and does not use any ionizing radiation (x-rays).

Why Am I Having this Test?

Your physician has ordered an MRI scan because it can provide more detailed and precise information than plain x-ray examinations for your condition. Magnetic resonance imaging is an extremely accurate method of disease detection throughout the body in areas such as the following:

- Head—stroke, brain injury (bleeding and swelling), tumor, infection, ruptured aneurysm, chronic disorders such as multiple sclerosis and Alzheimer's disease, and evaluation of the underlying cause of such symptoms as headaches, paralysis, dementia, altered sensation, and vision and hearing problems (Figs. 5-3, 5-4)
- Heart—anatomic and functional disorders of the heart muscle, chambers, and valves, coronary arteries, and aorta (aneurysm and dissection)
- Breast—evaluating questionable findings on mammography or ultrasound and assessing for possible rupture of a silicone breast implant (see p. 129)

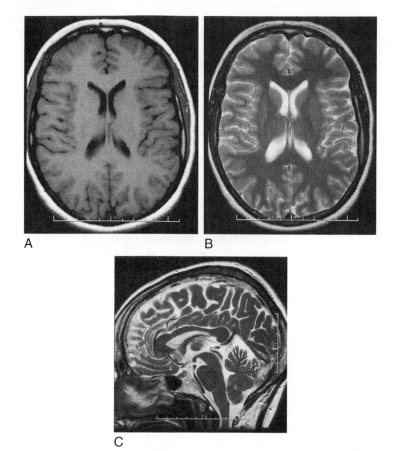

Figure 5-2. MRI of normal brain. (A) On a T1-weighted axial image, cerebrospinal fluid within the ventricles appears dark, while the white and gray matter appear as shades of gray. (B) On a T2-weighted image, the cerebrospinal fluid is white. (C) Sagittal T2-weighted image demonstrates the cerebral cortex, ventricles, pons, and cerebellum.

- Abdomen—tumors, cysts, or abscesses of the abdominal organs (liver, pancreas, spleen, kidneys, adrenals; Fig. 5-5); bile duct obstruction causing jaundice; and abnormalities of the pancreatic duct (Fig. 5-6)
- Pelvis—abnormalities of the uterus, ovaries, and fallopian tubes in women and of the prostate and seminal vesicles in men (Figs. 5-7, 5-8)
- Spine—herniated disc, spinal stenosis (narrowing of the spinal canal), spinal tumors and infection (Fig. 5-9), compression fractures, abnormalities of the spinal cord, and evaluation of symptoms of back pain and sciatica (Fig. 5-10)

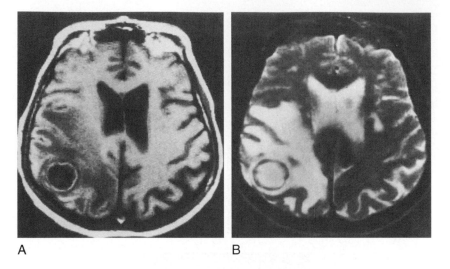

A   B

Figure 5-3. Brain abscess. (A) T1-weighted scan shows a central low-density, necrotic, infectious mass surrounded by low-signal-intensity edema. (B) On the T2-weighted image, the low intensity capsule is highlighted by increased signal centrally and peripherally.

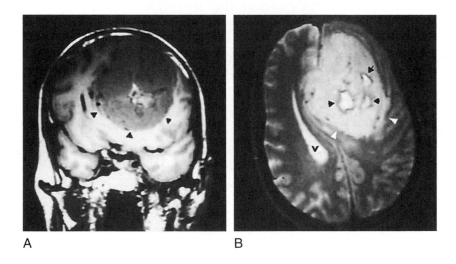

A   B

Figure 5-4. Meningioma. Huge mass (arrowheads) with low signal intensity on a T1-weighted coronal image (A) and high signal intensity on the T2-weighted axial image (B). Note the dramatic shift of the ventricle (v) caused by the mass effect of the tumor. The black arrows point to areas of hemorrhage within the tumor.

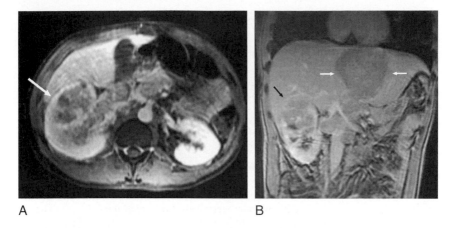

Figure 5-5. Renal cell carcinoma metastatic to the liver. (A) Axial image shows a large low-intensity mass on the right (arrow), which proved to be a carcinoma of the kidney. (B) On a coronal image, there is a large metastasis in the left lobe of the liver (white arrows) in addition to the renal mass (black arrow).

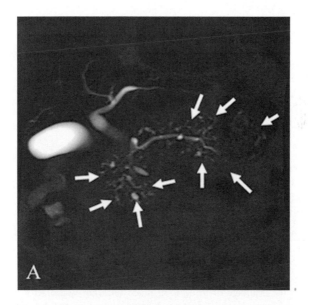

Figure 5-6. Pancreatic neoplasm. MRCP (magnetic resonance cholangiopancreatogram) demonstrates innumerable bright cystic lesions within the pancreas, which are connected to an otherwise normal main pancreatic duct.

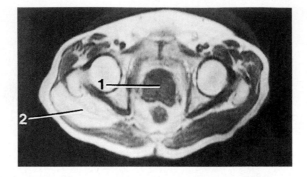

Figure 5-7. Benign prostatic hypertrophy. T1-weighted axial image shows generalized enlargement of the prostate gland with homogeneously low signal intensity (1). The large area of high signal intensity (2) in the right gluteal region represents a benign fatty tumor (lipoma).

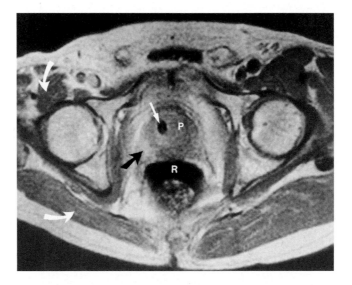

Figure 5-8. Carcinoma of the prostate. T1-weighted axial image demonstrates an abnormal area of increase signal intensity (black arrow) within the prostate gland (P). A Foley catheter for drainage of urine is in place (straight white arrow), and the rectum (R) contains air and feces. Note the decreased size of the pelvic muscles on the right (curved white arrows) in this patient with an above-the-knee amputation.

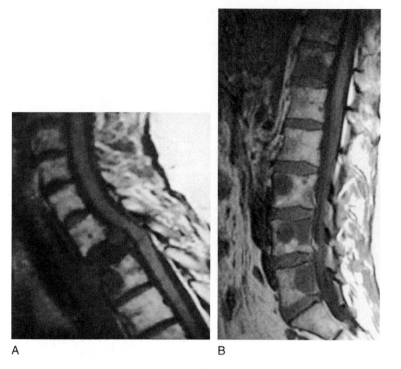

A   B

Figure 5-9. Spine metastases. (A) Lateral view shows gross tumor destruction and replacement of the body of T2, which has collapsed. On this sequence, the metastasis is darker than the normal vertebral marrow or the spinal cord, which is focally indented and displaced posteriorly by the tumor. There is also a lytic (dark) metastasis involving the anterior portion of T3. (B) In this patient with breast cancer, there are multiple lytic (dark) metastases throughout the lumbar spine.

- Extremities—detection of subtle fractures (Fig. 5-11), avascular necrosis (Fig. 5-12), arthritis, bone marrow abnormalities, and joint damage (to cartilage, menisci, tendons, and ligaments; Fig. 5-13)
- Blood vessels—see "Magnetic Resonance Angiography (MRA)" in Chapter 8

MRI also can be used for needle guidance during interventional procedures, such as tissue biopsy or drainage of an abscess, and for determining how far a cancer has spread (*staging* the tumor) (Fig. 5-14).

What Should I Tell My Doctor?

Before going for an MRI scan, make certain to tell your doctor if you:

- Are or may be pregnant or are breast feeding

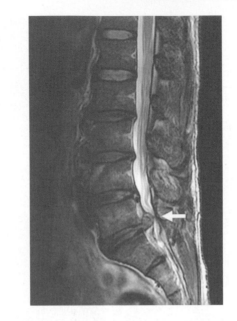

Figure 5-10. Herniated disc. Protrusion of the dark material of the disc (arrow) into the spinal canal was the cause of severe back pain in this patient.

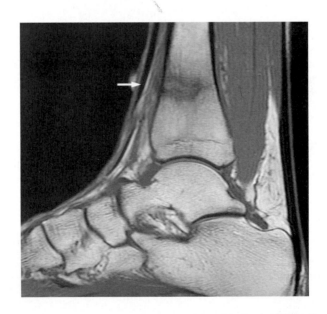

Figure 5-11. Stress fracture. The arrow points to edema (black area) in the distal portion of the tibia.

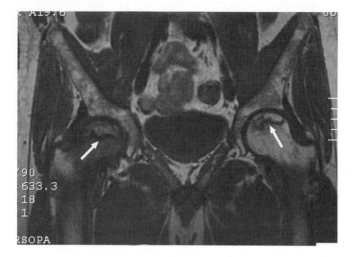

Figure 5-12. Avascular necrosis. Areas of abnormal bone marrow surrounded by a serpentine, irregular black line (arrows) in both femoral heads.

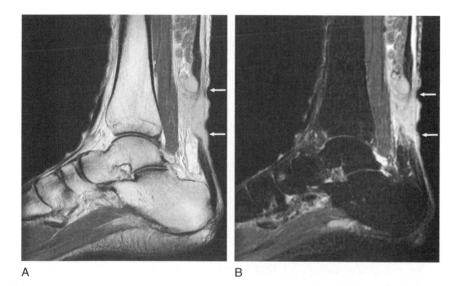

A   B

Figure 5-13. Achilles tendon rupture. (A) T1- and (B) T2-weighted sagittal images show a full thickness tear of the tendon with wide retraction of the proximal and distal fragments (arrows).

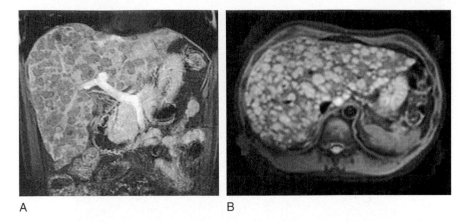

A   B

Figure 5-14. Liver metastases. (A) Numerous hypovascular metastases appear as dark areas within the liver. (B) On this diffusion-weighted image, the multiple metastases appear white.

- Are allergic to any medicine (unlike with CT, the contrast material used for MRI does not contain iodine)
- Have kidney disease that may prevent you from being given gadolinium, the most commonly used MRI contrast material
- Have an implanted medical device that uses electronics, such as a heart pacemaker or defibrillator, or an implanted infusion pump (such as an insulin pump for diabetes, a narcotics pump for pain medication, or a nerve stimulator for back pain)
- Have medical devices that contain metal, such as surgical clips (especially for brain aneurysm repair) and staples, artificial heart valves, vena cava filters, joint replacements, implanted spinal stabilization rods, tooth fillings and braces, metal stents, brain shunt tubes, or an intrauterine device (IUD); these devices may blur the images, but most of them do not preclude an MRI examination
- Wear a medication patch that contains metal
- Have an artificial limb
- Have a cochlear (ear) implant for hearing impairment
- Have retained metal in the eye socket (usually due to occupational exposure)
- Become nervous when in small spaces (claustrophobia); if so, you may need a sedative to relax and keep still (and you should arrange for someone to take you home after the procedure); note that this is less of a problem with "open" magnets

- Are unable to lie on your back for 30–60 minutes
- Weigh more than 300 pounds

Open magnets

Some individuals experience claustrophobia (fear of enclosed spaces) when surrounded by a traditional MRI unit. To address this problem, some equipment manufacturers have developed so-called open magnets, which have been designed so that the magnet does not completely surround the patient. Newer open MRI units produce high-quality images for many types of examinations. However, those using older magnets may have lower quality, and certain types of studies cannot be performed using open MRI equipment.

Why Was MRI Developed and How Does It Work?

Plain radiographs have two important limitations. First, it is impossible to display in a two-dimensional x-ray picture all the information contained in the three-dimensional area being examined. Objects in front of or behind the area of interest are superimposed, which may cause confusion unless side (lateral) or angled (oblique) views are taken. Second, conventional x-rays cannot distinguish among various soft tissues such as blood, nerves, or muscles, and among organs such as the liver, pancreas, and spleen, unless contrast material is used.

Unlike plain radiographs and CT, MRI does not use x-rays. Instead, it employs a strong magnetic field to align the protons of hydrogen atoms. Special wire coils placed around the part of the body to be imaged send a beam of radio waves of a specific frequency that cause the hydrogen atoms to absorb energy. Depending on the time required by the hydrogen atoms in specific tissues to return to their baseline state (relaxation time), faint signals are produced that are detected by the receiver portion of the coils, so that the patient is almost turned into an FM radio station. These signals are translated by a complex computer program into visual images that represent thin slices of the body. The radiologist can view these sections in varying angles on a television-like monitor.

Historical vignette

The early term for magnetic resonance imaging was *nuclear magnetic imaging* (NMR). However, in the mid-1980s, researchers decided to eliminate the word *nuclear*, with its unpopular public connotation. Consequently, the name was changed to the now universally accepted *magnetic resonance imaging* (MRI).

How Do I Prepare for an MRI Scan?

The key to preparation for an MRI scan is to remember that metal objects are *not* allowed in the examination room and should be left at home if possible. In rare cases, a large metallic object can cause severe injury if it flies through the air at great speed toward the magnet. Objects that should not be taken into the room with the magnet include:

- Jewelry, watches, credit cards with magnetic strips, and hearing aids (can be damaged by the strong magnetic field)
- Pins, hairpins, and metal zippers (can distort the MRI images)
- Removable dentures
- Eyeglasses, pens, and pocket knives
- Body piercings

If you do bring any metal objects with you, they must be removed before the MRI scan and placed in a secured locker, which is available to store personal possessions.

In general, MRI is safe for patients with most metal implants (such as heart valves), though you should always make certain that your physician is aware of them before ordering the study. You also should mention such implants to the MR technologist (or radiologist) before entering the MR scanning area. However, if you have the following implants, you should *not* go into the room where the MR examination is performed unless explicitly instructed to do so by a radiologist or technologist who is aware that you have one of them:

- Internal (implanted) heart pacemaker or defibrillator
- Implanted infusion pump (such as an insulin pump for diabetes, a narcotics pump for pain medication, or a nerve stimulator for back pain)
- Cochlear (ear) implant
- Some types of surgical clips used to clamp off brain aneurysms

In general, metal objects used in orthopedic surgery (pins, screws, plates, or surgical staples) pose no risk during MRI. However, a recently placed artificial joint (hip, knee) may require the use of another imaging procedure. If there is any question, an x-ray image can be obtained to determine whether you have a metallic object in your body. Similarly, a preliminary x-ray may be needed if you have a tattoo (some contain iron and could heat up during an MRI) or a history of an accident, or if you have worked around metal that could have resulted in some tiny fragments lodged around your eye.

For an abdominal MRI scan, you may be asked not to eat or drink for several hours before the examination. Unless you are told otherwise, you may follow your normal diet and routine and take medications as usual. If you will require a sedative to relax during the procedure, you should arrange for someone to drive you home after the test.

What Does the Equipment Look Like?

An MRI scanner consists of three parts, two of which you will actually see. The machine itself is a large, cylindrical tube surrounded by a circular magnet that looks somewhat like a huge doughnut and contains the magnet and detectors (Fig. 5-15). You will be placed on a movable examination table that slides in and out of the center of the magnet. The third part of the scanner is the sophisticated computer that processes all the imaging information; it is located in a separate room.

There are two other major magnet configurations. *Short-bore* systems are designed so that you are not completely surrounded by the magnet; *open* magnets are open on all sides. These units are especially helpful for examining claustrophobic patients who are fearful of being in a closed space and for those who are very obesc and do not fit in the standard MRI machine.

How Is the Test Performed?

When you arrive at the radiology imaging department or facility, you may be asked to remove some or all of your clothing (especially anything with

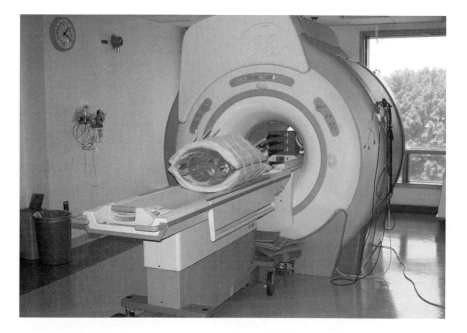

Figure 5-15. MRI scanner with dedicated abdominal coil positioned on the sliding table.

metal fasteners) and change into a lightweight gown to wear during the examination. If you are allowed to keep some of your clothes on, you will be asked to empty your pockets of all coins and cards with scanner strips (such as ATM and credit cards), since the MRI magnet may erase the information on them.

You will be asked to lie down on the movable examination table that slides into the middle of the magnet. Bolsters and straps may be used to support you and help you to maintain the proper position during the study. If you are overly anxious inside the MRI magnet, you may be given a sedative to make you more relaxed so that you can remain motionless.

Small devices that contain coils capable of sending and receiving radio waves may be placed around or adjacent to the area of the body to be scanned. A special belt strap may be used to sense your breathing or heartbeat, triggering the machine to take the images at the proper time.

If contrast material will be used in your MRI exam, a nurse or technologist will insert an intravenous (IV) line into a vein in your hand or arm. A saline solution will drip through the IV to keep the line open until the contrast material is injected after the initial series of scans. Additional images will be taken following the injection.

When the MR images are being obtained, you will hear loud, repetitive clicking and humming noises that may sound like machine gun fire. You may be given ear plugs or headphones with music to reduce the noise. Magnetic resonance imaging examinations generally include multiple runs (sequences), some of which may take several minutes to perform. During this time, it is very important that you lie completely still and breathe normally to prevent blurring of the images. At times, you may be asked to hold your breath for short periods.

The technologist will leave the MRI room and go to the control room while the examination is being performed. However, the technologist will always be able to see you through the control-room window and will be in voice contact with you via a two-way intercom system throughout the test (Fig. 5-16). Some facilities permit a parent or friend to stay in the room.

The scanning time for an MRI exam depends on the area of the body studied and the number of sequences required. It usually takes about 30–60 minutes but can last as long as 2 hours. When the examination is completed, you may be asked to wait until the technologist checks the images to determine whether additional sequences are needed. If you have received IV contrast material, the line will be removed. There is no required recovery period after an MRI examination. Once the study is over, you are free to leave the radiology department or facility and resume your normal diet and activities.

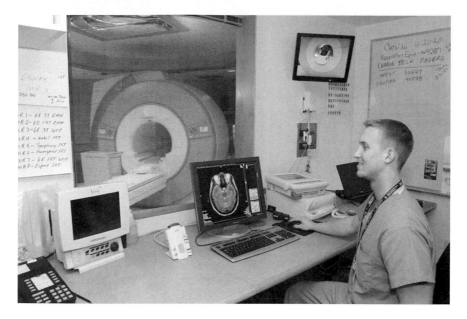

Figure 5-16. MRI control room with the technologist continually able to see the table and magnet through a window.

What Will I Feel?

Most MRI examinations are painless, and you will not feel any effect from the magnetic field or the radio waves. You may find it uncomfortable to remain still during the procedure or experience a sense of being closed in (claustrophobia). Remember that sedation can be arranged if you think you will be overlying anxious, but fewer than 1 in 20 patients actually requires it. If you have metal dental fillings, you may feel a tingling feeling in your mouth.

You will always know when images are being obtained because you will hear the loud tapping or thumping sounds when the coils generate the radio-frequency pulses. Each sequence may take a few seconds to a few minutes. You will be able to relax between the imaging sequences, but you should maintain your position as much as possible. After the procedure is over, you may feel tired or sore from lying in one position for a long time on the hard table. The room may feel cool because of the air conditioning needed to protect the sensitive machinery.

For some types of MRI examinations, you will be asked to hold your breath for a few seconds. Remember that it is normal for the area of your body being imaged to feel slightly warm. If it feels hot, notify the technologist. If you receive contrast material, it is normal to feel coolness and flushing for a minute or two. A few patients experience nausea or an allergic reaction of hives or itchy eyes. The IV needle may cause you some discomfort when it is inserted, and you may feel some bruising when it is removed.

It is recommended that nursing mothers not breast feed for 24 hours after an MRI exam with a contrast material.

What Are the Advantages and Disadvantages of MRI Compared with CT?

Advantages

- Noninvasive imaging technique that does not involve exposure to ionizing radiation (x-rays)
- No known harmful effects from the strong magnetic fields used
- Higher spatial and soft-tissue contrast resolution and the possibility of dynamic scanning
- Use of multiple sequences can reduce artifacts and precisely identify and characterize structural abnormalities throughout the body
- Able to directly image in multiple planes without the need to reformat the images
- Imaging modality of choice for evaluating the central nervous system (including the brain and spinal cord) and the musculoskeletal system (including joints and the spine)
- Permits evaluation of the biliary tree and pancreatic ducts noninvasively and without contrast injection
- The contrast material used in MRI (gadolinium) is less likely to cause an allergic reaction than the iodine-based materials used for CT scanning and catheter angiography (though it can be dangerous in patients with pre-existing kidney disease)
- May be used in pregnant women since, unlike CT, it involves no ionizing radiation (Fig. 5-17); however, although there is no reason to believe that MRI harms the fetus, pregnant women usually are advised not to have this study unless it is medically necessary

Disadvantages

- Longer procedure and more expensive than CT
- The powerful magnet used in MRI prevents it from being used if the patient has an internal (implanted) heart pacemaker or defibrillator, an implanted infusion pump (such as an insulin pump for diabetes, a narcotics pump for pain medication, or a nerve stimulator for back pain),

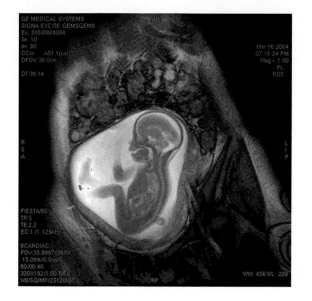

Figure 5-17. MRI in pregnancy. The fetus is well seen in this profile view.

or a cochlear (ear) implant; some types of surgical clips used to clamp off brain aneurysms; or metal fragments near the eye (a preliminary plain x-ray may be required to exclude this)
- Complications: the powerful magnet may stop a nearby watch; erase information on ATM and credit cards; pull any loose metal objects toward it (possibly causing injury); and cause iron pigments in tattoos or tattooed eyeliner to produce skin or eye irritation or a burn from some medication patches
- In people with poor kidney function, high doses of MRI contrast material have been associated with a very rare but possibly serious condition called *nephrogenic systemic sclerosis*
- Claustrophobia from the need to lie for a prolonged period in a closed area inside the magnetic tube
- Loud noise produced during the examination
- Inability to demonstrate the outer margin (cortex) of bone for showing fractures, though it superbly depicts the bone marrow
- Requires the patient to lie perfectly still for up to several minutes (CT scans take only a few seconds)
- Although extremely sensitive to the detection of abnormalities, MRI may be less able to provide a specific diagnosis; for example, in an

MRI study of the head, an identical high signal intensity on T2-weighted images can be produced by such widely different conditions as infarction (stroke), tumor, infection, and demyelinating disease (such as multiple sclerosis)

MR Arthrography

What Is MR Arthrography?

Arthrography is an imaging study in which contrast material is injected directly into a joint to evaluate its structure and function. It provides valuable information about joint abnormalities and can help determine whether there is a need for surgical correction or even joint replacement. Today arthrography is combined with MRI for optimal visualization of the internal structures of a joint, such as the articular cartilage, joint capsule, tendons, ligaments, and surrounding muscles. Magnetic resonance arthrography is most commonly performed in the shoulder and knee, though the hip, ankle, wrist, and temporomandibular joints may also be evaluated with this technique.

Why Am I Having this Test?

An MR arthrogram is used to discover the cause of unexplained pain, swelling, or limited range of motion of a joint. Your physician may also order an MR arthrogram if your clinical symptoms suggest:

- Rotator cuff tear or frozen shoulder (Fig. 5-18)
- Cruciate or collateral ligament damage or loose bodies in the knee
- Abnormal fluid-filled cysts or neoplastic growths related to a joint

Arthrography using fluoroscopy (without MRI) can be used to confirm that a thin needle has been placed correctly before a sample of joint fluid is removed for analysis, to check needle placement before the injection of a painkiller such as a corticosteroid, and to assess for possible loosening of a joint replacement.

What Should I Tell My Doctor?

Before going for an MR arthrogram, make certain to tell your doctor if you:

- Are or suspect that you may be pregnant
- Are allergic to gadolinium, the contrast material used in this procedure
- Have any of the devices that might prevent you from having an MRI (see p. 102)

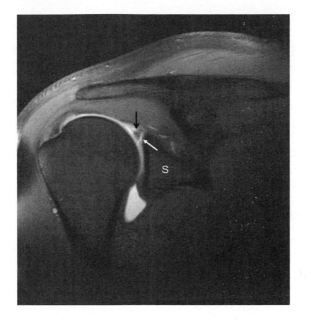

Figure 5-18. MR arthrogram of the right shoulder. The patient has a so-called SLAP (superior labrum, anterior to posterior) tear, with the superior labrum identified with the black arrow. Contrast material injected into the shoulder joint extends into the tear (white arrow), making it more conspicuous.

Why Was MR Arthrography Developed and How Does It Work?

A plain radiograph shows only the bones that articulate to form a joint. However, it cannot demonstrate the cartilage lining the outside of the bones; the tendons, ligaments, and joint capsule that stabilize it; or the surrounding muscles that permit the joint to function. To visualize optimally the anatomy of these structures and their function, it is necessary to image the joint after the injection of contrast material directly into it. Known as *arthrography,* the procedure initially used iodinated contrast material, with the images obtained under x-ray fluoroscopy. The development of MRI allowed high-quality imaging of the internal structures of a joint without any contrast injection. However, certain joints and the specific disorders involving them are better evaluated using MR arthrography, which combines these two techniques to provide exquisite anatomic detail that may permit detection of abnormalities not seen on conventional MR. Unlike traditional arthrography, the contrast material used in MR arthrography contains no iodine and has a lower risk of complications.

How Do I Prepare for an MR Arthrogram?

There is no special preparation; however, no metal object can be brought into the examination room (see p. 132).

What Does the Equipment Look Like?

Because MR arthrography is a composite of two different procedures, you will first have the needle inserted into your joint under fluoroscopy (see p. 31) and then images will be made in the MR suite.

How Is the Test Performed?

For the first part of the procedure, you will lie down on a table in a fluoroscopy room. The skin around the joint will be cleaned with an antiseptic soap, and a local anesthetic will be injected into the area. After the area is numb, a needle will be placed into the joint space under fluoroscopic control. When the needle is in the correct place, any joint fluid will be drained and sent to the laboratory for analysis. After contrast material is injected into the joint, the needle will be removed to prevent the contrast from escaping. You will be asked to move the joint through its entire range of motion so that the contrast material is distributed throughout the joint space. This part of the examination is usually completed in about 30 minutes.

You will then be taken to the MRI scanner for a series of images of the affected joint. Depending on the number of sequences obtained, this part of the study may take as long as 45 minutes.

After the MR arthrogram is completed, you may leave the imaging department or facility. You should rest the joint for about 12 hours and refrain from any strenuous activity for 1–2 days. Apply ice to the area if there is any swelling and take an over-the-counter pain medicine if necessary. If a bandage or wrap is placed on the joint following the procedure, you will be told when you can remove it.

Complications of MR arthrography are uncommon. You should call your physician immediately if you experience:

• Significant joint pain for more than 1–2 days
• Any sign of infection (fever, chills, red streaks or pus related to the puncture site)
• Continued bleeding or increasing swelling at the puncture site

What Will I Feel?

You will feel a pinprick and momentary burning when the local anesthetic is given. When the contrast material is injected, you may experience some fullness in the joint and hear a gurgling sound when the joint is moved. After the examination, you may have some mild pain, tenderness, stiffness, and swelling in the joint and hear some unusual clicking, cracking, or grating sounds when you move the joint. All of these feelings are normal and should disappear within about 24–48 hours.

What Are the Advantages and Disadvantages of MR Arthrography?

Advantages

- Optimal procedure for visualizing the internal structure of a joint and the surrounding tissues and for determining whether a surgical procedure or even joint replacement is required
- No iodinated contrast material is required

Disadvantages

- More expensive and time-consuming than conventional arthrography performed under fluoroscopy
- As with all arthrography, a slight chance of complicating infection or bleeding in the joint

6

BREAST IMAGING

Mammography

What Is Mammography?

Mammography is an x-ray examination. It uses low-energy x-rays to produce an image of the breast that aids in the early detection and diagnosis of cancer and other diseases of the breast in women.

Based on population averages, it is estimated that about one in eight women born today will be diagnosed with breast cancer at some point during their lives. The most important risk factor for breast cancer is age. Most breast cancers occur in women over age 50, and the disease is relatively uncommon in women under 40.

Why Am I Having this Test?

Your health care provider has ordered a mammogram because it is the best way to find abnormalities in the breast before they can be felt. This procedure also can be useful in explaining the cause of symptoms (such as a lump) relating to your breast. There are two different types of mammograms—screening and diagnostic.

A *screening* mammogram is used to detect breast changes in women who have no signs or symptoms of breast cancer. It is designed to identify tumors that are too small to feel, as well as to demonstrate microcalcifications (tiny calcium deposits in the breast) that sometimes indicate the presence of breast cancer (Fig. 6-1). Screening mammograms are often read by the radiologist after the patient has left the radiology department or office.

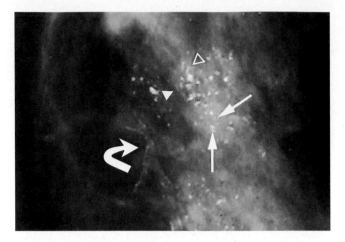

Figure 6-1. Screening mammogram. Numerous tiny calcifications with linear (straight arrows), curvilinear (solid arrowhead), and branching (open arrowhead) forms are characteristic of malignancy. Note the benign calcification in the arterial wall, which it easily recognized by its large size and tubular shape (curved arrow).

According to the National Cancer Institute, women without breast symptoms who are at average risk for breast cancer should have a screening mammogram every 1–2 years beginning at age 40. Women who are at higher than average risk for breast cancer (see below) should talk with their health care providers about whether to have their first screening mammogram before age 40 and how often to have follow-up examinations. Recently, a government-sponsored task force (2010) proposed a highly controversial new screening regimen, which would eliminate mammograms for women under age 50, provide mammograms only every other year for women between ages 50 and 74, and stop all breast cancer screening in women over 74.

A *diagnostic* mammogram is ordered when there is a specific problem or condition that needs to be addressed. It may be requested if you have:

- A lump that can be felt (Fig. 6-2)
- A sign or symptom of breast cancer such as pain, skin thickening, nipple discharge, or a change in breast size or shape
- A possible abnormality suggested on a screening mammogram that requires additional images for full evaluation (Fig. 6-3)
- A finding on a previous mammogram that is being monitored
- Implants that make it difficult to evaluate the breast on standard screening views

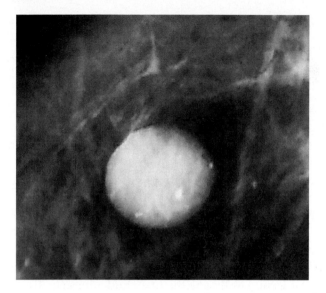

Figure 6-2. Diagnostic mammogram for a palpable lump. The smooth, round with clearly defined margins represents a benign fibroadenoma.

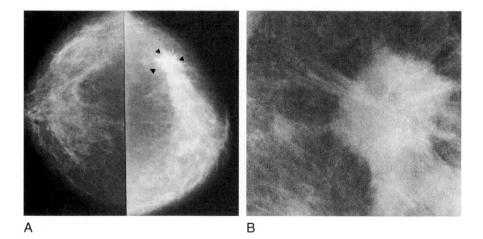

A   B

Figure 6-3. Breast cancer. (A) The initial screening mammogram shows an irregular mass (arrows). (B) A magnified and coned diagnostic mammogram well demonstrates the ill-defined, irregular mass with radiating spicules, an appearance that is characteristic of malignancy.

What Are the Factors that Increase the Risk of Breast Cancer?

The risk of breast cancer increases gradually as a woman gets older. However, the following factors are associated with a higher likelihood of developing this disease:

- A personal history of breast cancer (women who have had one breast cancer are more likely to develop a second)
- A family history of breast cancer (in a mother, sister, or daughter, especially if it was diagnosed before age 50)
- Specific breast changes on biopsy (atypical hyperplasia, lobular carcinoma *in situ*)
- Genetic abnormalities (specific alterations in certain genes, such as *BRCA1* and *BRCA2*)
- Abnormal reproductive and menstrual history (beginning menstruation before age 12 or experiencing menopause after age 55, as well as never having had a child or having the first child after age 30)
- Long-term use of hormone therapy after menopause (using combination estrogen-progestin hormone therapy for more than 5 years)
- Radiation therapy to the chest (including the breasts) before age 30
- Use of diethylstilbestrol (DES), a medication that was given to some pregnant women in the United States between 1940 and1970
- Increased body weight (overweight or obese after menopause)
- Decreased level of physical activity
- High levels of alcohol consumption

What Should I Tell My Doctor?

Before going for a mammogram, make certain to tell your doctor if you:

- Are or may be pregnant, or have delivered a baby within the past 6 months
- Are breast feeding or have stopped breast feeding within the past 6 months
- Are experiencing any breast symptoms such as a lump, pulling in (retraction) of the nipple, nipple discharge, skin discoloration or dimpling.

Why Was Mammography Developed and How Does It Work?

Early detection of breast cancer offers the opportunity for more effective treatment and the greatest chance for cure. Mammography was developed to detect breast cancers before they can be felt. The breasts consist of fat, glandular tissue, and fibrous tissue, all of which look similar on regular x-rays.

To overcome this limitation, x-ray equipment was developed specifically for breast imaging. These mammography machines use lower-energy x-rays and special x-ray film that permits the very fine-detail images required to detect small abnormalities.

More recently, digital mammography equipment has been developed. Unlike conventional mammogram machines that produce images on film (like a traditional camera), digital units (like digital cameras) take electronic images that are stored directly in a computer and can be read on a monitor. The recorded data can be magnified, enhanced, and otherwise manipulated to improve detection of abnormalities in the breast. In addition, digital mammography decreases the number of repeat images (reducing radiation exposure) and permits long-distance consultations with other specialists in the field. However, from the point of view of the patient, there is essentially no difference between these two types of mammographic procedures.

Another new development is the use of computer-aided detection (CAD). Using digitized mammographic images, which can be obtained from either a conventional film mammogram or one that is digitally acquired, sophisticated computer software searches for abnormal areas of density, mass, or calcification that may indicate the presence of breast cancer. The CAD system highlights these areas on the images, alerting the radiologist to the need to re-examine them for possible abnormalities.

What Is the MQSA?

To ensure that mammograms are safe and reliable, the federal government passed the Mammography Quality Standards Act (MQSA), which requires all mammography facilities in the United States to meet stringent quality standards, be accredited by the Food and Drug Administration (FDA), and be inspected annually. These stringent standards apply to the technologist who takes the mammogram, the radiologist who interprets it, and the medical physicist who tests the mammography equipment. All mammography facilities are required to display their FDA certificate, and you should make certain that it has not expired. The MQSA regulations also require mammography facilities to give patients an easy-to-read report on the results of their mammogram.

How Do I Prepare for a Mammogram?

You will be given a gown and asked to undress from the waist up. Wearing a two-piece outfit will make changing easier. Large necklaces can get in the way of the mammogram, so you may be asked to remove them. You should not use any powder, deodorant, or creams under your arms or under you breasts on the day of the mammogram, since these can sometimes show up on the pictures and raise questions. If you have used any of these items, let the technologist who is doing the mammogram know and you will be given the opportunity to clean off your skin. You can bring deodorant with you to apply after the mammogram is completed.

The breasts are squeezed during the mammogram in order to get the best picture possible. Some women find this compression very uncomfortable. If you still get your period, you can try to schedule the mammogram for a time during the menstrual cycle when your breasts are least tender, usually during the first half of the monthly cycle. In addition, some women find that taking an over-the-counter medication such as aspirin, ibuprofen, or acetaminophen an hour before the test decreases the discomfort.

If you have had a previous mammogram at another site, it is very important to bring the prior films with you. Having older mammograms for comparison improves the accuracy of the reading. Remember that it is the images themselves that must be compared; this cannot be done based on the written report. If your previous studies are not available for comparison, the interpretation of your mammogram could be delayed. At times, it could mean that you will need to have additional pictures that may not have been necessary if the older mammograms were supplied.

What Does the Equipment Look Like?

A mammography machine is a rectangular box, roughly the size of a refrigerator, that houses the tube that produces the x-rays. Attached to the unit are two plates that hold and compress the breast to obtain the best possible images (Fig. 6-4). The part of the apparatus that takes the image can be turned 360° in order to obtain pictures at different angles.

How Is the Test Performed?

Mammography is performed as an outpatient procedure. Before the test begins, you probably will be asked to fill out a form providing information about your medical history. You will be asked if you are currently having any breast problems; if there is any history of breast cancer in your family; your reproductive history (including the age when you first got your period; how many children, if any, you have; how old you were when you had your first child; whether you are still having your period and, if so, the date of your last period; and whether you are taking hormones); and whether you have had any breast surgery or needle biopsies in the past.

You will be standing when the x-ray pictures are taken (Fig. 6-5). For a screening mammogram, two views of each breast are taken at different

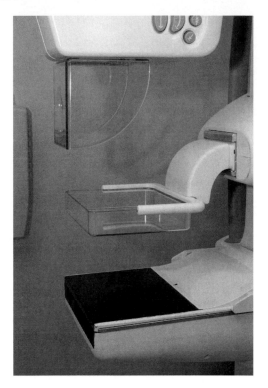

Figure 6-4. Mammography machine with compression device.

angles, for a total of four pictures. For a diagnostic mammogram, the number of pictures and the angles at which they are taken vary, depending on the reason that the mammogram is being done. For each picture, the breast is squeezed between two plates, one of which records the x-ray image. The reason for compressing the breast is to separate out overlapping tissue to give a clearer picture. Squeezing the breast makes the tissue thinner, so that less radiation is needed to produce the image; this also decreases the chance of movement while the picture is being taken, which could cause blurring.

You will be asked to hold your breath, again to minimize motion, while the picture is being taken. Each image takes only a few seconds to produce. A screening mammogram is usually completed in a few minutes. The pictures are checked by the technologist for technical quality and, if they are adequate, you are done. Repeat views are sometimes required, usually because there is some blurriness due to motion or because not enough breast tissue is included in the image.

In general, screening mammograms are read by the radiologist after you have left the radiology department or facility. If there is a questionable finding that requires more images or ultrasound, you will be contacted to return

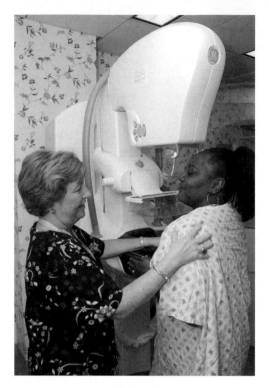

Figure 6-5. Patient in the upright position for a mammogram.

for these additional tests. This occurs about 10% of the time after a screening mammogram, but it is less frequent if there are previous mammograms for the radiologist to use for comparison. For diagnostic mammograms, the images are first checked for technical quality by the technologist and you will be asked to wait until they are reviewed by the radiologist. If any additional pictures are needed, they are obtained before you leave.

What Will I Feel?

Because the breasts are squeezed by the compression paddle to obtain clearer pictures with a minimum of radiation, you may feel discomfort or even pain if your breasts are particularly sensitive. You may feel tugging as the technologist pulls your breasts away from your chest in order to include as much tissue in the image as possible. The positioning may feel awkward and uncomfortable, but it is important to remember that each image takes only a few seconds to complete and that good positioning results in better pictures. The x-rays themselves cannot be felt.

How Do I Get the Result of My Mammogram?

Within 30 days of mammography, you will be notified in writing of the results by the department or facility where the test was done. The notification is often in the form of a letter that is written in plain (not medical) language. If you have had a diagnostic mammogram, the radiologist who interprets the study or the technologist who performed it will sometimes give you the results before you leave the facility. If you have had a screening mammogram and there is a finding that requires more testing to decide whether it is important, you will be contacted by either the radiology office or the doctor who sent you for the mammogram, usually well before 30 days. If you have any questions about the results of your mammogram, you should discuss them with your doctor or with the radiologist. If you have not received any results by 30 days, you should contact the facility where you had the mammogram and ask about them.

What Are the Benefits and Risks of Mammography?

Benefits

- Improves the detection of small cancers in the breast before they can be felt. Many large studies have shown that when women have screening mammography, the death rate from breast cancer is decreased by about 25%.
- Provides more information about the cause of a breast symptom, such as a lump that can be felt
- Years of extensive experience have indicated which findings on mammography need more attention and which are not worrisome
- Noninvasive study that does not require needles or injections
- Relatively inexpensive and usually covered by insurance
- Readily available, relatively fast, and easy to perform

Risks

- Radiation exposure—Since mammography is an x-ray procedure, there is a theoretical risk of causing cancer. However, this risk is extremely small, especially since the breasts are less sensitive to radiation as a woman gets older. Moreover, the possible benefit of finding an early cancer at a curable stage far outweighs any radiation risk.
- False-positive results—After a screening mammogram, about 10% of women are called back for more mammographic images (a diagnostic mammogram) or ultrasound to look more closely at a questionable finding. Most often, these added views or ultrasound will indicate that

there is nothing wrong, with the suspicious area representing either overlapping normal tissue or a harmless cyst. If any question persists after the additional testing, a biopsy may be recommended. It is important to keep in mind that most biopsies are benign.

• False negative results—Like any other diagnostic test, mammography is not perfect and some cancers cannot be seen. A small tumor may be hidden in dense breast tissue, especially in younger women. If a lump can be felt, a negative mammogram does not necessarily mean that there is no problem, and further testing may be necessary. However, mammography should be the first step in evaluating a breast symptom because it can often provide important information about the cause.

• Overdiagnosis—There is an argument that mammography sometimes detects a cancer that would never have grown to be life-threatening. This means that some women who have mammographic screening for breast cancer undergo unnecessary treatment. Unfortunately, there is no way of knowing which early cancers that have not spread outside the breast will become aggressive. The likelihood of this theoretical risk is unknown, but it is probably not a common occurrence. It is important to remember that mammographic screening has been proven to save lives, with the death rate from breast cancer dropping in this country along with the increased use of screening mammography.

• Finding cancer does not always mean saving lives—Even though mammography can identify tumors that cannot be felt, this may not help a woman with a fast-growing or aggressive cancer that has already spread to other parts of the body before being detected.

Breast Ultrasound

What Is Breast Ultrasound?

Ultrasound is a test that uses high-frequency sound waves to produce a picture of the tissues of the breast. Because sound waves rather than x-rays are used, ultrasound provides different information from that obtained by mammography. For example, fluid and solid tissue look identical on mammograms, but ultrasound can differentiate between them. Dense breast tissue, which can hide lumps on mammography, does not interfere with ultrasound. In general, breast ultrasound is used as an addition to mammography rather than as a replacement for it. Mammograms will detect abnormalities that are not seen on ultrasound and vice versa.

Why Am I Having this Test?

Your doctor has ordered a breast ultrasound examination to get more information about your breasts. Some of the reasons for having breast ultrasound include:

- Getting more information about a suspicious area seen on a mammogram
- Determining the cause of a symptom such as a beast lump, an area of thickening, or a nipple discharge
- Screening for breast cancer in women who have dense, thick breast tissue that might hide lumps on mammography
- Obtaining information about a lump that can be felt in a pregnant or very young woman who should not have a mammogram because of the risk of radiation

What Should I Tell My Doctor?

- If you are having any breast symptoms
- The date of your last mammogram and the results (if your doctor is not aware of them)

Why Was Breast Ultrasound Developed and How Does It Work?

The breast is made up of fat, glandular, fibrous, and connective tissues, which are found in various proportions in different women. Some women normally have very dense breasts, which limits the ability of mammography to detect abnormalities within them but does not pose any problem for ultrasound. In addition, a malignant mass and a benign cyst may appear identical on mammography. Because sound waves travel differently through liquid and solid tissue, ultrasound is an excellent way of distinguishing a fluid-filled cyst from a tumor (Figs. 6-6, 6-7).

Ultrasound imaging uses high-frequency sound waves, which cannot be heard by the human ear, to produce an image of structures inside the body. A transducer (probe) pressed against the skin sends out small pulses of high-frequency sound waves, which reflect off organs, fluids, and tissues within the body and return to a sensitive microphone within the transducer. By measuring these echo waves, the ultrasound machine can determine the size and shape of each body structure, how far away it is from the source of the sound, and whether it is solid, filled with fluid, or contains both. A computer instantly transforms this material into real-time black-and-white or color moving images on the monitor. A technologist then takes individual still pictures that can be interpreted by the radiologist.

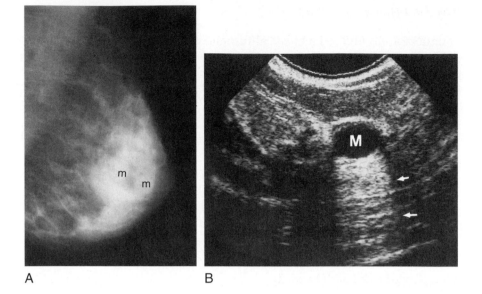

A   B

Figure 6-6. Ultrasound of benign breast cyst. (A) Initial mammogram shows several rounded masses (m), which could be solid or cystic, in a breast that is very dense anteriorly. (B) Sonogram clearly demonstrates that the largest mass (M) has no internal echoes and shows considerable posterior enhancement (arrows), features that are diagnostic of a benign cyst.

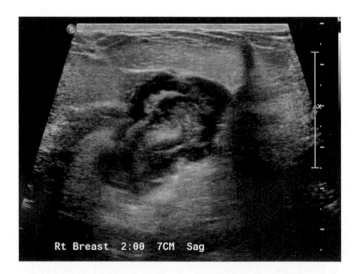

Figure 6-7. Ultrasound of breast abscess. Sonogram in a woman who was breast feeding demonstrates an ill-defined complex cyst with solid (light) and cystic hypoechoic (dark) elements and low-level internal echoes, consistent with an abscess.

How Do I Prepare for Breast Ultrasound?

No specific preparation is necessary for breast ultrasound. The use of deodorant and powder, which is discouraged before having a mammogram, does not interfere with breast ultrasound. You will be given a gown and asked to undress from the waist up, so wearing a two-piece outfit will make changing easier.

What Does the Equipment Look Like?

An ultrasound scanner consists of a computer and a video display screen with a small hand-held transducer that sends and receives the sound waves through the tissues.

How Is the Test Performed?

After having undressed from the waist up and put on a gown, you will be asked to lie on your back or roll slightly onto one hip, with the arm on the side to be examined raised above your head. In most cases, the ultrasound examination is performed by a technologist (sonographer), who is supervised by a radiologist. A clear, warmed gel is spread on the portion of the breast being studied so that the transducer can make secure contact and eliminate air pockets between it and the skin that would degrade the image. The sonographer or radiologist then presses the transducer firmly against the skin and sweeps it back and forth over the area of interest while viewing a picture of the underlying tissues on a video monitor. You may be asked to change positions for additional scans to be made.

You may be having an ultrasound examination of one or both breasts. If the test is being performed for screening, all areas of both breasts will be studied. If it is being done to get more information about a mammographic finding or a lump that can be felt, only a limited area of the breast will be examined.

How long a breast ultrasound examination takes depends on whether both breasts or merely a limited area of one breast is being examined. Generally, the entire ultrasound examination is finished within 15–30 minutes. Once the imaging is completed, the technologist will wipe the gel off your skin and you can resume your normal activities.

What Will I Feel?

Most ultrasound examinations are painless and fast. You will not hear or feel the sound waves. The gel spread on your skin may feel cold unless it is first warmed to body temperature. You will feel light pressure from the transducer as it passes over your breast, and you may experience some discomfort if you have an area that is tender.

What Are the Benefits and Risks of Breast Ultrasound?

Benefits

- Generally painless
- No radiation
- Accuracy is not affected by dense breast tissue
- Usually can differentiate between a harmless fluid-filled cyst in the breast and a solid growth that might need more attention
- Often provides added information about findings seen on mammography or about a palpable breast lump
- Can be used to guide needle biopsy of a breast lump

Risks and Disadvantages

- Only demonstrates the area directly under the transducer, so small abnormalities elsewhere in the breast can be missed
- False negatives—Ultrasound does not detect some abnormalities that can be seen on mammography (especially small calcifications that may be the sign of early breast cancer). Therefore, ultrasound should *not* be used to replace mammography but only in addition to it (except in pregnant or very young women, who should not be exposed to ionizing radiation).
- False positives—Some apparent abnormalities detected by breast ultrasound turn out to be nothing, but they must be biopsied to be certain.

Breast MRI

What Is Breast MRI?

Magnetic resonance imaging is a noninvasive test that uses a powerful magnetic field and pulses of radio wave energy to make detailed pictures of organs and other structures inside the body. In some cases, the unique features of MRI allow this technique to provide different information about suspected breast abnormalities than mammography and ultrasound.

At times, MRI can detect breast abnormalities that cannot be seen with any other imaging procedure.

Why Am I Having this Test?

Your physician has ordered this test because it can sometimes give more detailed and precise information about the breasts than other tests, such as mammography or ultrasound. Some of the circumstances in which breast MRI has been shown to be useful include:

- Evaluating whether silicone breast implants are ruptured (Fig. 6-8)
- Determining the extent of disease in a woman who has just been diagnosed with breast cancer
- Further evaluating a questionable finding on a mammography, ultrasound, or physical examination (Fig. 6-9)
- Screening for breast cancer in women who are at high risk (see p. 118)

What Should I Tell My Doctor?

Before going for an MRI examination, make certain to tell your doctor if you:

- Are or may be pregnant or are breast feeding
- Are allergic to any medicine (unlike CT, the contrast material used for MRI does not contain iodine)
- Have kidney disease that may prevent you from being given gadolinium, the most commonly used MRI contrast material

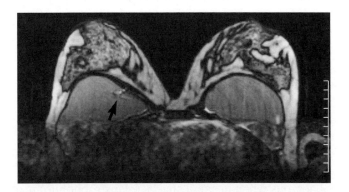

Figure 6-8. MRI of breast implants. This technique can distinguish between breast tissue (upper) and the implant (lower) and show that there is no evidence of rupture. The arrow points to a small fold in the implant.

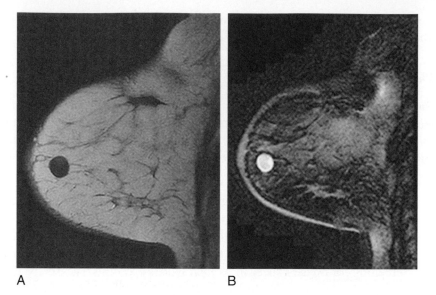

A   B

Figure 6-9. MRI of benign breast cyst. Mammography and ultrasound were equivocal in this patient. MRI shows a well-defined, round mass that demonstrates characteristic findings of a benign cyst filled with protein or hemorrhage, with low signal on a T2-weighted image (A) and high signal on a T1-weighted scan (B).

- Have an implanted medical device that uses electronics, such as a heart pacemaker or defibrillator, or an implanted infusion pump (such as an insulin pump for diabetes, a narcotics pump for pain medication, or a nerve stimulator for back pain)
- Have medical devices that contain metal, such as surgical clips (especially for brain aneurysm repair) and staples, artificial heart valves, vena cava filters, joint replacements, implanted spinal stabilization rods, tooth fillings and braces, metal stents, brain shunt tubes, and an intrauterine device (IUD); these may blur the images, but most of them do not preclude an MRI examination
- Wear a medication patch that contains metal
- Have an artificial limb
- Have a cochlear (ear) implant for hearing impairment
- Have retained metal in the eye socket (usually due to occupational exposure)
- Become nervous when in small spaces (claustrophobia); if so, you may need a sedative to relax and keep still (and should arrange for someone to take you home after the procedure); note that this is less of a problem with open magnets

- Are unable to lie on your back for 30–60 minutes
- Weigh more than 300 pounds

Why Was Breast MRI Developed and How Does It Work?

Mammography and ultrasound are the two imaging techniques that are generally used to evaluate the breast. However, both of these tests have limitations. First, it is impossible to display in a two-dimensional x-ray picture all the information contained in the three-dimensional area being examined. Objects in front of or behind the area of interest are superimposed, which may cause confusion. Dense breast tissue interferes with the ability of x-rays to see abnormalities on mammograms. Ultrasound is not affected by dense breast tissue, but this test often cannot detect very small abnormalities and will miss abnormalities that are not included in the pictures that are generated.

Magnetic resonance imaging employs a strong magnetic field to align the protons of hydrogen atoms. Special wire coils placed around the part of the body to be imaged send a beam of radio waves of a specific frequency that cause the hydrogen atoms to absorb energy. Depending on the time required by the hydrogen atoms in specific tissues to return to their baseline state (relaxation time), faint signals are produced that are detected by the receiver portion of the coils, so that you are effectively almost turned into an FM radio station. These signals are translated by a complex computer program into visual images that represent thin slices of the body. The radiologist can view these sections in varying angles on a television-like monitor and can even see three-dimensional images.

In the breast, MRI has been shown to be effective in detecting small abnormalities that may not be felt or seen with mammography or ultrasound.

How Do I Prepare for a Breast MRI?

The key to preparation for MRI is to remember that metal objects are *not* allowed in the examination room and should be left at home if possible. In rare cases, a large metallic object can cause severe injury if it flies through the air at great speed toward the magnet. Objects that should not be taken into the room with the magnet include:

- Jewelry, watches, credit cards with magnetic strips, and hearing aids (can be damaged by the strong magnetic field)
- Pins, hairpins, and metal zippers (can distort the MRI images)
- Removable dentures

- Eyeglasses, pens, and pocket knives
- Body piercings

If you do bring any metal objects with you, they must be removed before the MRI scan and placed in a secured locker that is available to store personal possessions.

In general, MRI is safe for patients with most metal implants (such as heart valves), though you should always make certain that your physician is aware of them before ordering the study. You also should mention them to the MR technologist (or radiologist) before entering the MR scanning area. However, if you have the following implants, you should *not* go into the room where the MR examination is performed unless explicitly instructed to do so by a radiologist or technologist who is aware that you have one of them:

- Internal (implanted) heart pacemaker or defibrillator
- Implanted infusion pump (such as an insulin pump for diabetes, a narcotics pump for pain medication, or a nerve stimulator for back pain)
- Cochlear (ear) implant
- Some types of surgical clips used to clamp off brain aneurysms

In general, metal objects used in orthopedic surgery (pins, screws, plates, or surgical staples) pose no risk during MRI. However, a recently placed artificial joint (hip, knee) may require the use of another imaging procedure. If there is any question, an x-ray image can be obtained to determine whether you have a metallic object in your body. Similarly, a preliminary x-ray may be needed if you have a tattoo (some tattoos contain iron and could heat up during an MRI) or a history of an accident, or if you work around metal and there is a possibility that some tiny fragments are lodged around your eye.

For breast MRI, you may follow your normal diet and routine and take medications as usual. If you will require a sedative to relax during the procedure, you should arrange for someone to drive you home after the test.

If you are still getting your period, it is best to have breast MRI during the second week of your cycle (days 10 to 14 after you start your period) to decrease the possibility of a false-positive reading. However, if you have a medical need for an urgent MRI, it is not absolutely necessary to wait until the second week of your cycle to have the study done.

What Does the Equipment Look Like?

An MRI scanner consists of three parts, two of which you will actually see. The machine itself is a large, cylindrical tube surrounded by a circular magnet that looks somewhat like a huge doughnut. You will be placed on a movable examination table that slides into and out of the center of the magnet. The third part of the MRI scanner is the sophisticated computer that processes all the imaging information; it is located in a separate room.

How Is the Test Performed?

Magnetic resonance imaging can be performed as an inpatient or outpatient. When you arrive at the radiology imaging facility, you may be asked to remove some or all of your clothing (especially anything with metal fasteners) and change into a lightweight gown to wear during the examination. If you are allowed to keep some of your clothes on, you will be asked to empty your pockets of all coins and cards with scanner strips (such as ATM and credit cards), since the MRI magnet may erase the information on them.

You will be asked to lie on your stomach on the movable examination table that slides into the middle of the magnet. Your breasts will be hanging in a special holder called a *breast coil*. Bolsters and straps may be used to help you remain still and in the proper position during the study. If you are overly anxious while inside the MRI magnet, you may be given a sedative so that you can relax and can keep still.

All breast MRI examinations are done with IV contrast except those done to determine if silicone implants are ruptured. If contrast material will be used in your MRI exam, a nurse or technologist will insert an IV line into a vein in your hand or arm before you enter the scan room. Once you are positioned on the scanning table, preliminary scans will be obtained and then the contrast injected. Additional images will be taken following the injection.

When the MR images are being obtained, you will hear loud, repetitive clicking, knocking, and humming noises that may sound like machine gun fire. You will be given ear plugs or headphones with music to reduce the noise. Magnetic resonance imaging examinations generally include multiple runs (sequences), some of which may take several minutes to perform. During this time, it is very important that you lie completely still and breathe normally to prevent blurring of the images.

The technologist will leave the MRI room and go to the control room while the examination is being performed. However, the technologist will always be able to see you through the control-room window and will be in voice contact with you via a two-way intercom system throughout the test.

The scanning time for a breast MRI is usually about 30–60 minutes. When the examination is completed, you may be asked to wait until the technologist checks the images to determine if additional sequences are needed. If you have received IV contrast material, the line will be removed. There is no required recovery period after an MRI examination. Once the study is over, you are free to leave the radiology facility and resume your normal diet and activities.

What Will I Feel?

Most MRI examinations are painless, and you will not feel any effect from the magnetic field or the radio waves. You may find it uncomfortable to remain still during the procedure or experience a sense of being closed in (claustrophobia). Sedation can be arranged if you think that you will be overlying anxious, but fewer than 1 in 20 patients actually requires it. If you have metal dental fillings, you may feel a tingling feeling in your mouth.

You will always know when images are being obtained because you will hear loud tapping or thumping sounds when the coils generate the radio-frequency pulses. Each sequence may take a few seconds to a few minutes. You will be able to relax between the imaging sequences, but you should maintain your position as much as possible. After the procedure is over, you may feel tired or sore from lying in one position for a long time on the hard table. The room may feel cool because of the air conditioning needed to protect the sensitive machinery.

It is normal for the area of your body being imaged to feel slightly warm. If it is very uncomfortable, notify the technologist. If you receive contrast material, it is normal to feel coolness and flushing for a minute or two. Rarely, patients will experience nausea or an allergic reaction of hives or itchy eyes. The IV needle may cause some discomfort when it is inserted, and you may have some bruising when it is removed.

It is recommended that nursing mothers not breast feed for 24 hours after an MRI with contrast material.

What Are the Advantages and Disadvantages of MRI Compared with Mammography or Breast Ultrasound?

Advantages

- Noninvasive imaging technique that does not involve exposure to radiation
- No known harmful effects from the strong magnetic fields used
- Can detect breast abnormalities, including cancers, that may not be seen on either mammography or ultrasound
- Unlike mammography, accuracy is not affected by dense breast tissue
- Unlike breast ultrasound, MRI provides a full picture of the breast that does not depend on the skill of the person producing the pictures

Disadvantages

- MRI is a longer and more expensive procedure than mammography and ultrasound. Insurance companies sometimes require prior authorization before they will pay for breast MRI, and sometimes the claim is denied.
- False positives—Although MRI can detect very small abnormalities that mammography and ultrasound might miss, it may suggest abnormalities that turn out to be unimportant. This can lead to additional testing and even an unnecessary biopsy.
- The powerful magnet used in MRI prevents this study from being used if you have an internal (implanted) heart pacemaker or defibrillator, an implanted infusion pump (such as an insulin pump for diabetes, a narcotics pump for pain medication, or a nerve stimulator for back pain), a cochlear (ear) implant, some types of surgical clips used to clamp off brain aneurysms, or metal fragments near the eye (a preliminary plain radiograph may be required to exclude this).
- Complications of the powerful magnet—The magnet may stop a nearby watch, erase information on ATM and credit cards, pull any loose metal objects toward it (possibly causing injury), or cause iron pigments in tattoos or tattooed eyeliner to produce skin or eye irritation, or a burn from some medication patches containing metal.
- In people with poor kidney function, high doses of MRI contrast material have been associated with a very rare but possibly serious condition called *nephrogenic systemic sclerosis.*
- Claustrophobia from the need to lie a closed area inside the magnetic tube; loud noises produced during the examination

Breast Biopsy

What Is a Breast Biopsy?

Lumps and other breast abnormalities are often detected by physical examination, mammography, or other imaging studies. However, it is not always possible to tell from these imaging tests whether a growth is benign or cancerous. To make a precise diagnosis, a breast biopsy may be performed to remove tissue from a suspicious area in the breast and examine it under a microscope. This may be done surgically or through a less invasive procedure involving a hollow needle placed in the breast under mammographic (stereotactic), ultrasound, or MRI guidance. It must be remembered that image-guided needle biopsy is not designed to remove the entire abnormality, but merely to obtain a large enough tissue sample to make the diagnosis.

Why Am I Having a Breast Biopsy?

A breast biopsy may be indicated if prior imaging procedures have demonstrated such suspicious abnormalities as:

- A mass that is not a simple cyst
- An area of distortion in the structure of the breast tissue
- An area of abnormal tissue change, including worrisome calcifications

There are various types of imaging-guided biopsy. These include:

- Fine needle aspiration (FNA)—insertion of a tiny needle (smaller than one used to draw blood) to extract fluid or cells from the abnormal area
- Core-needle biopsy—use of a large, hollow needle to remove one sample of breast tissue on each insertion
- Vacuum-assisted device—use of a vacuum-powered instrument that uses pressure to collect multiple tissue samples during one needle insertion
- Wire localization—placement of a thin guide wire into the suspicious area to localize the lesion for a subsequent surgical biopsy

What Should I Tell My Doctor?

Prior to a needle biopsy, you should tell your doctor about all medications that you are taking, including herbal supplements, and if you have any allergies, especially to anesthesia. As with any interventional procedure, inform your doctor if you are or may be pregnant.

How Do I Prepare for a Breast Biopsy?

Your physician probably will advise you to stop taking aspirin or a blood thinner up to a week before the procedure. Even if you will not be sedated, try to arrange for a relative or friend to drive you home after the biopsy.

How Is a Breast Biopsy Performed?

Minimally invasive procedures such as stereotactic, ultrasound- or MRI-guided breast biopsy are usually performed on an outpatient basis by a specially trained radiologist. For a breast biopsy using ultrasound guidance, you will be asked to lie on your back on the examination table or turned slightly to the side. Conversely, for stereotactic or MRI-guided biopsy, you will lie face down with the affected breast positioned in an opening in the table (Fig. 6-10). For MRI-guided biopsy, the table is movable and an IV

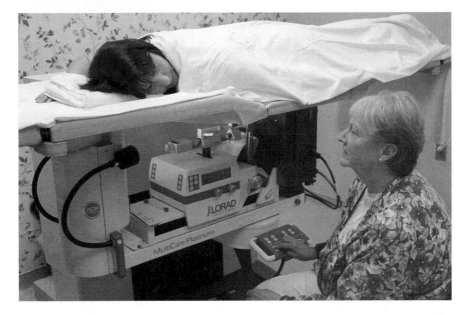

Figure 6-10. Stereotactic table for performing breast biopsy under mammographic guidance.

line will be inserted in a vein in your hand or arm to inject contrast material (just as when the diagnostic MRI was done). A local anesthetic will be injected into the breast to numb it before the biopsy needle is inserted. Tissue samples will be obtained by one of the three methods mentioned above (Fig. 6-11). Often a tiny localizing clip is placed in the breast at the end of the procedure to mark the spot that was biopsied and, if needed, to assist in finding it again. The clip is nonallergic and cannot be felt. Once the biopsy is complete, the needle will be removed and pressure applied to stop any bleeding. The opening in the skin will be covered with a dressing; no sutures are needed. The entire procedure is usually completed within 45–60 minutes.

What Will I Feel?

You will be awake during a breast biopsy and should have little or no discomfort. You may feel a stick and some burning when the needle is inserted and the local anesthetic is injected to numb the breast. There may be some pressure when the biopsy needle is inserted. For most women, the major discomfort from the procedure is the need to lie or their stomach or back for up to an hour.

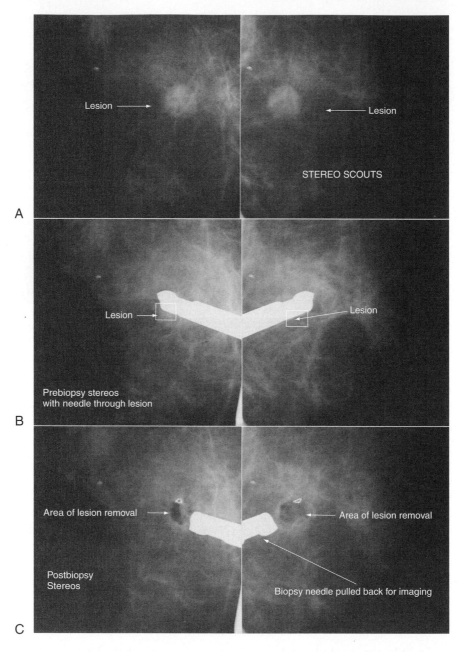

Figure 6-11. Stereotactic needle biopsy. (A) Scout images of a breast mass. (B) Needle localization. (C) Post-biopsy images with the needle pulled back demonstrate removal of the mass.

Some transient bruising, tenderness, or minimal bleeding following a breast biopsy is normal. However, you should contact your physician if you have severe pain, an enlarging breast, or bleeding that worries you. If you stopped taking any medicine to have the biopsy done, you should stay off it for another 3 days. Also, avoid strenuous activity for 3 days after returning home; after that time, you should be able to resume your normal activities.

What Are the Advantages and Disadvantages of Imaging-Guided Breast Biopsy Compared with Surgical Biopsy?

Advantages

- Less invasive and leaves little or no scarring
- Shorter procedure (usually completed in less than an hour)
- Rapid recovery time

Disadvantages

- Image-guided breast biopsies may occasionally miss a lesion or underestimate its extent. If the diagnosis remains uncertain after a breast biopsy performed under ultrasound or MRI guidance, a surgical biopsy is usually required.
- Infrequent complications of image-guided biopsy include bleeding and infection

7

NUCLEAR MEDICINE

Nuclear Medicine

What Is Nuclear Medicine?

Nuclear medicine is a branch of medical imaging that uses small amounts of radioactive isotopes (radionuclides, or tracers) to diagnose or treat various diseases. Unlike most other imaging modalities, nuclear medicine tests demonstrate the physiologic function rather than the anatomy of the body system being investigated. At times, nuclear medicine images can be superimposed on anatomic studies such as CT or MRI to provide information about both the structure and function of specific organs and tissues in the body. Nuclear medicine also can be used for therapeutic purposes, such as the use of radioactive iodine (I-131) to treat cancer and other medical conditions of the thyroid gland.

Why Am I Having this Test?

Radionuclide imaging is used to demonstrate the function and structure of organs and systems throughout the body. Your physician may order this as a diagnostic procedure if your clinical symptoms suggest:

- Fracture, infection, metastatic cancer, arthritis, or avascular necrosis (bone scan)
- Pulmonary embolus obstructing blood flow (lung scan)
- Abnormal blood flow to the heart or abnormal cardiac function (myocardial perfusion scan)
- Overactive or underactive thyroid function (thyroid uptake and scan)

- Bleeding into the bowel (labeled red blood cell scan)
- Infection of unknown source (labeled white blood cells or a Ga-67 scan)

What Should I Tell My Doctor?

Before going for a radionuclide scan, make certain to tell your doctor if you:

- Are or might be pregnant.
- Are breast feeding (if so, use formula and discard your breast milk for 1–2 days after the scan until the radioactive tracer has been eliminated from your body)
- Have within the past 4 days had an x-ray procedure using barium contrast material (such as an upper GI series or a barium enema) or have taken a medicine that contains bismuth (such as Pepto-Bismol), because barium and bismuth can interfere with test results.

Why Was Nuclear Medicine Scanning Developed and How Does It Work?

Plain radiographs demonstrate structural abnormalities of various parts of the body but provide only indirect evidence of their function. Nuclear medicine studies use tiny amounts of radioactive materials that are injected into a vein, swallowed, or inhaled as a gas and eventually accumulate in different organs and tissues. These tracers give off small amounts of energy in the form of gamma rays, which can be detected by special cameras to produce computerized images that can be interpreted by a radiologist. Unlike a plain radiographic examination, in which x-rays pass through your body, are absorbed to various degrees by structures within it, and then produce an image on a recording device on the other side of the body, in most nuclear medicine scans the source of the radiation is within your own body and travels to the surface, where it is detected by the gamma camera.

Unlike other imaging techniques, nuclear medicine imaging studies are primarily designed to show physiologic processes within the body, such as blood flow and rates of metabolism and cellular activity. Areas of greater intensity, called *hot spots*, indicate sites where large amounts of the radiotracer have accumulated and there is a high level of chemical activity. Less intense areas, or *cold spots*, represent smaller concentrations of radiotracer and less chemical activity.

Radioactive substances decay at a predictable rate that is specific for each radioactive nucleus. This property is usually described as the *half-life*—the time required for the radioactive material to decay to half of the initial amount.

How Do I Prepare for a Nuclear Medicine Scan?

There is no special preparation for a nuclear medicine scan. You can eat and drink whatever you like. However, you should consider limiting your fluid intake for several hours before the test, because you will be asked to drink extra fluids after the radioactive tracer is injected to help flush it from your body in the urine. Bring something to read or do if you are having one of the nuclear medicine scans (such as a bone scan or myocardial perfusion imaging) that require you to wait for several hours after the injection before the images are taken.

What Does the Equipment Look Like?

Most nuclear medicine procedures are performed using a gamma camera (Fig. 7-1), which contains one or more large, flat, rectangular sodium iodide

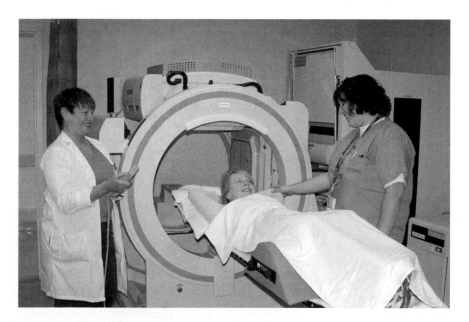

Figure 7-1. Gamma camera.

crystals that detect the gamma rays emitted from the radionuclide tracer within your body. The gamma camera may be suspended over the examination table from a tall, movable post, be part of a metal arm that hangs over the table, or rotate around your body. In single photon emission tomography (SPECT) and positron emission tomography (PET) scanners, the detector system rotates around the patient and is situated within a large doughnut-shaped machine that is similar in appearance to a CT scanner. A sophisticated computer system, often located in an adjacent room, processes all of the imaging information and transforms it into an image that can be seen on a television-like monitor.

How Is the Test Performed?

Nuclear medicine scans may be performed on an inpatient or outpatient basis. Depending on the area being examined, you may be asked to remove all or most of your clothes (you may be able to keep on your underwear) and will be given a lightweight gown to wear. The radioactive tracer will be injected into a vein in your arm, swallowed, or inhaled as a gas. The period of time required for the radioactive tracer to travel through your body and accumulate in the organ being studied can range from a few seconds to several days. Consequently, the actual scanning may begin immediately or be delayed for a few hours or even several days. If the scan is not performed soon after the radionuclide has been given, you usually will be allowed to leave the radiology facility until it is time for the scan to be done. Depending on the type of nuclear medicine examination, the actual scanning time may vary from less than 30 minutes to several hours and may take place over several days.

During the scanning, you initially will lie on your back while the gamma camera or SPECT/PET device takes a series of images. These may be focused on a small area, such as the heart or lungs, or include your entire body from head to toe (as in a bone scan). You may be asked to assume different positions so that the area of interest can be viewed from various angles. During each scan, you must stay very still to get the highest-quality pictures and avoid blurring the images. For some nuclear medicine examinations, a small handheld probe is passed over the area of the body being studied to measure levels of radioactivity. Other studies measure radioactivity levels in your blood, urine, or breath. You may be asked to drink several glasses of water to eliminate in your urine any of the radioactive material that has not accumulated in the area of interest.

After the nuclear medicine scan has been completed, you may be asked to wait for a few minutes until the technologist checks the images to make certain that no additional scanning is needed. Then you are free to leave the radiology facility and resume your normal activities. The radioactive tracer used in most nuclear medicine procedures is a short-lived isotope (technetium-99m) that has a half-life of only 6 hours. Therefore, it will be completely eliminated from your body within 2 days. You will be instructed to drink a large amount of fluid and empty your bladder frequently for 1–2 days after the procedure to help flush the remaining radionuclide from your body. It is important to remember that you do not pose a hazard to other people, since the tracer emits less radiation than a standard x-ray study.

What Will I Feel?

Most nuclear medicine procedures are completely painless. If the radioactive tracer is injected intravenously, you will feel a slight pinprick as the needle goes through your skin. When the radionuclide is injected, you should not experience any discomfort. Swallowed radionuclides have little or no taste. Inhaling radionuclides in gaseous form should feel no different from breathing room air. For most people, the most difficult part of the test is lying on the back (or in some other position) without moving while the scan is being made. Ask the technologist for a pillow or blanket to make yourself as comfortable as possible before the actual scanning begins.

In certain instances, usually after receiving treatment doses of radioactive iodine, you may be instructed to take special precautions after urinating, such as flushing the toilet twice and washing your hands thoroughly, since most of the administered dose will be excreted into your urine.

What Are the Advantages and Disadvantages of Nuclear Medicine Studies?

Advantages

- Provides unique information that cannot be obtained by other imaging techniques
- Offers information about physiologic function and cellular activity
- Less expensive than cross-sectional studies such as CT and MRI
- Painless and minimally invasive (intravenous line)
- Low radiation exposure
- Allergic reactions to radioactive tracers are rare

Disadvantages

- Time-consuming (it may take hours or days for the radiotracer to accumulate in the part of the body being studied, and the imaging process itself may take several hours to perform)
- Poor resolution of anatomic structures compared to other imaging techniques (especially CT and MRI)
- Although often highly sensitive for detecting an abnormality, radionuclide imaging may be less able than other techniques to make a specific diagnosis. For example, a hot spot on a bone scan could represent a fracture, infection, benign bone tumor, or metastasis (focus of spread from a malignant tumor).
- More expensive than plain radiographs

Special Types of Nuclear Medicine Studies

Bone Scan

A bone scan is a nuclear medicine test that detects areas of abnormal bone mineral resorption or deposition. Areas of rapid bone growth or repair absorb a large amount of an intravenously administered radioactive tracer and appear on images as bright or hot spots that may indicate the presence of arthritis, fracture (Fig. 7-2), infection, or tumor, or such bone lesions as fibrous dysplasia and Paget's disease. Conversely, areas that absorb little or no tracer appear as dark or cold spots, which may indicate decreased blood flow to the bone (infarction or avascular necrosis).

One of the most common reasons for a bone scan is to detect the spread of cancer to bones (metastases). Because cancer cells multiply rapidly and have increased cellular activity (metabolism), metastases appear as multiple hot spots of increased radioactivity (Fig. 7-3). Bone scanning is highly sensitive for detecting the presence of metastases or other bony abnormalities, often demonstrating them long before they can be seen on plain radiographs. However, the bone scan often cannot determine the specific cause of these findings. Therefore, areas of suspected metastases or other abnormalities are often further examined by plain radiographs, CT, or MRI. The bone scan also can be used to evaluate other causes of bone pain, such as a fracture that is not evident on a plain x-ray study.

For most bone scans, you will be asked to wait for 2–4 hours after the injection of the radionuclide until enough of it has been absorbed by your bones for an image to be obtained. During this time, you may leave the radiology facility. If the bone scan is being performed to determine whether you have an infection (osteomyelitis), images will be taken as the radioactive

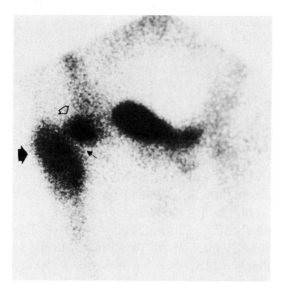

Figure 7-2. Stress fracture. Radionuclide bone scan shows greatly increased uptake in the femoral neck (open arrow) and intertrochanteric region (solid arrow), with lack of uptake at the actual fracture site (thin arrow). Plain radiographs showed only very subtle changes.

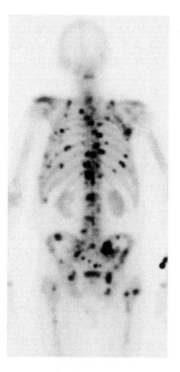

Figure 7-3. Metastases to bone. Screening radionuclide bone scan in a patient with newly diagnosed prostate carcinoma demonstrates multiple focal areas of abnormal isotope uptake (black areas) throughout the skeleton.

tracer is injected, shortly after the injection, and then 3–4 hours later when it has collected in the bones. A scan of the entire skeleton takes about 1 hour; scanning limited to a specific part of the body requires less time.

Lung Scan

A lung scan is most commonly used to detect a pulmonary embolism, a blood clot that prevents normal blood flow to part of a lung. There are two types of lung scan—ventilation and perfusion—that are usually done together. In a ventilation lung scan, a radioactive tracer or mist is inhaled into the lungs. Images show areas of the lungs that are receiving too little air and appear dark (cold) or that are retaining too much air and appear bright (hot). For a perfusion lung scan, a radioactive tracer is injected into a vein in the arm and travels through the bloodstream to the lungs. If there is normal blood flow, images show an even distribution of radionuclide throughout both lungs. Areas of abnormal blood flow due to a pulmonary embolism appear as dark (cold) regions (Fig. 7-4). In the evaluation of a possible pulmonary embolism, ventilation and perfusion scans are usually performed together (V/Q scan), with the ventilation scan done first. If the lungs are working normally, blood flow on a perfusion scan matches air flow on a ventilation scan. A mismatch between the ventilation and perfusion scans may indicate the presence of a pulmonary embolism.

A plain chest radiograph is usually obtained soon before or shortly after the lung scan. The reason is that abnormal areas on both the ventilation and perfusion scans may represent underlying chest disease, such as pneumonia or pleural effusion (rather than pulmonary embolism), which can be clearly seen on a plain chest radiograph.

A ventilation scan takes about 15–30 minutes. A mask is placed over your mouth and nose. An alternative method is to place a clip on your nose and have you breathe through a tube in your mouth. You will be asked to inhale the tracer gas or mist through the mask or tube by taking a deep breath and then holding it. The gamma camera will make pictures by detecting radiation released by the tracer as it moves through your lungs. You may be asked to breathe the gas in and out through your mouth for several minutes. At times, you may be asked to hold your breath for about 10 seconds and to change positions so that your lungs can be viewed from other angles. After the procedure has been completed, the radioactive gas or mist is rapidly removed from your lungs as you breathe normally.

For a perfusion scan, images are taken after the intravenous injection of radioactive tracer. You will again be asked to assume different positions, usually on your side and stomach, so that your lungs can be viewed from different angles. The perfusion scan also takes about 15–30 minutes.

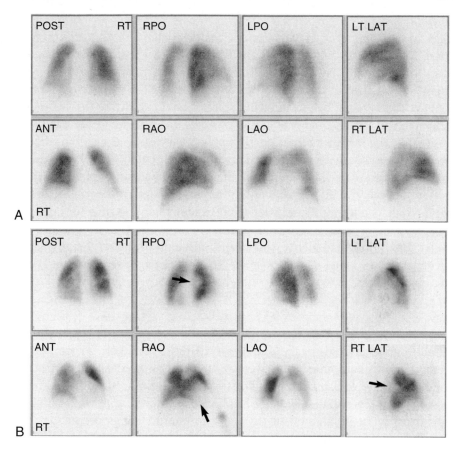

Figure 7-4. Pulmonary embolism. (A) Top two lines show a normal radionuclide perfusion scan with uniform isotope uptake in both lungs. (B) Bottom two lines from another patient show multiple wedge-shaped areas without isotope uptake (arrows), diagnostic of pulmonary emboli.

Thyroid Scan and the Radioactive Iodine Uptake Test

The thyroid scan and the radioactive thyroid uptake test (thyroid uptake) are nuclear medicine studies that provide information about the structure and function of the thyroid. This gland, located in the anterior neck just below the Adam's apple, controls the rate at which the body converts food to energy (metabolism). It makes and stores essential hormones that help regulate heart rate, blood pressure, and body temperature. The thyroid scan assesses the size, shape, and function of the gland, while the thyroid uptake test evaluates its function.

Thyroid scan

The thyroid scan is used to determine the size, shape, and position of the thyroid gland. The thyroid gland absorbs and concentrates iodine, which it uses to make hormones. The thyroid scan can be obtained after the oral ingestion of a small amount of radioactive iodine or the IV injection of technetium-99m pertechnetate, which also is taken up by the thyroid gland. The actual scanning time is about 30 minutes or less, though the total time you will spend in the imaging department will vary, depending upon whether oral or IV radioactive tracer is used.

The thyroid scan can demonstrate the size of the gland in patients with a goiter or overactive thyroid (hyperthyroidism) and determine whether a thyroid nodule is hot (highly radioactive and usually benign) or cold (no radioactivity within it and possibly malignant) (Fig. 7-5). A thyroid scan also can be used to follow up patients with cancer of the thyroid after therapy and to locate thyroid tissue outside the neck (such as at the base of the tongue or the upper chest).

Thyroid uptake test

A radioactive thyroid uptake test measures the amount of radioactivity in your thyroid gland after you have swallowed a small dose of radioactive iodine in liquid or capsule form. The thyroid gland absorbs iodine to make hormones; therefore, the amount of radioactive thyroid in the thyroid gland correlates with the amount of thyroid hormone that it is producing. The thyroid gland in a hypothyroid patient takes up too little iodine; a person with hyperthyroidism has an overactive gland that takes up too much iodine.

Many foods and medicines containing iodine can affect the results of a thyroid uptake test. These include iodized salt, kelp, seaweed, cough syrups, multivitamins, and the heart medicine amiodarone (Cordarone, Pacerone), as well as thyroid hormones and antithyroid hormones. Therefore, it is important that your doctor is aware of the names and doses of all of your medicines, both prescription and over-the-counter, before you have a thyroid uptake test. Your doctor will let you know if you need to stop taking any of them before the test. A recent imaging examination using contrast material that contains iodine or any radioactive material also can affect the results of a thyroid uptake test.

Before a thyroid uptake test, you may have a test that measures the amount of thyroid hormones (thyroid stimulating hormone[TSH], T3, T4) in your blood. The thyroid uptake test is usually obtained 4–6 or 24 hours (or both) after you swallow the radioactive iodine. Two separate uptake measurements are often made, each one requiring 5–10 minutes.

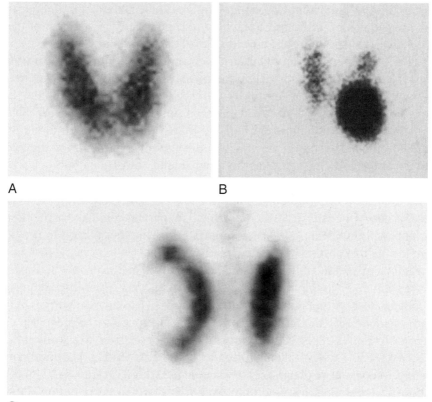

A   B

C

Figure 7-5. Thyroid scan. (A) Normal. There is uniform distribution of radionuclide activity throughout the entire gland. (B) "Hot" nodule. The highly radioactive area represents a benign mass. (C) "Cold" nodule. The area of the gland that is devoid of radioactive uptake, corresponding to the patient's palpable mass, represented a thyroid carcinoma.

Radioactive iodine therapy

Radioactive iodine (I-131) can be used to treat an overactive thyroid gland (hyperthyroidism). This condition can be caused by Graves' disease, in which the entire thyroid gland is hyperactive, or be due to one or more overactive nodules in the thyroid gland that are producing an excessive amount of thyroid hormone.

After the dose of I-131 is swallowed, it is absorbed through the gastrointestinal tract into the bloodstream and concentrated in the thyroid gland. There it destroys most or all of the thyroid cells, including those that are hyperactive or malignant. In patients with hyperthyroidism, symptoms of the disease resolve slowly, beginning about 2 weeks after treatment. The maximum benefit usually occurs at 3–6 months. Because the hormones produced by the thyroid are essential for regulating cellular activity throughout the body, most patients will need to take thyroid pills daily for the rest of their lives to ensure that they have a normal level of thyroid hormones.

After I-131 therapy, you can return home but should follow some precautions. Nearly all of the radioactive iodine leaves the body during the first 2 days following treatment, primarily through the urine. Small amounts are excreted in saliva, sweat, tears, vaginal secretions, and feces. To spare others from exposure to radiation, during this time you should sleep alone and avoid prolonged, close contact with other people, particularly pregnant women and small children. Launder your linens, towels, and clothes separately each day at home. Use private toilet facilities (if possible) and flush twice after each use. Bathe daily and wash your hands frequently. Use disposable eating utensils or wash your utensils separately from those of others. Patients with infants at home should arrange for another person to provide care for the first several days after treatment.

Radioactive iodine therapy should never be used in a woman who is pregnant, lest it damage the thyroid gland of the fetus. Many facilities require a pregnancy test within 24 hours before giving I-131 to any woman of childbearing age unless she has had a prior surgical procedure to prevent pregnancy. Most physicians recommend that I-131 not be given to a woman who is breast feeding unless she is willing to stop breast feeding her child completely. Many believe that pregnancy should be delayed at least 6–12 months following I-131 therapy, since the ovaries receive some radiation during treatment.

For up to 3 months after I-131 therapy, the level of radiation in your body may be sufficient to trigger the sensitive radiation detection devices used at airports and federal buildings. Therefore, you may want to ask your physician to provide a letter of explanation that you can carry with you.

Radioactive iodine therapy is also used to treat thyroid cancer by destroying malignant cells in the gland. In many cases, surgery is initially performed to remove as much of the cancerous tissue as possible. A whole-body thyroid scan is usually performed to identify any tumor metastases. Radioactive iodine is then given to destroy any remaining thyroid tissue and to kill any cancer cells that have spread to lymph nodes or other parts of the body. Radioactive iodine therapy is effective against any differentiated thyroid cancers (papillary, follicular) that absorb and concentrate iodine, but it is not used to treat undifferentiated (anaplastic) and medullary thyroid cancers that do not demonstrate any thyroid uptake.

Cardiac Scan

Cardiac nuclear medicine studies provide pictures of the structure and function of the heart to diagnose the cause of chest pain that is unexplained or

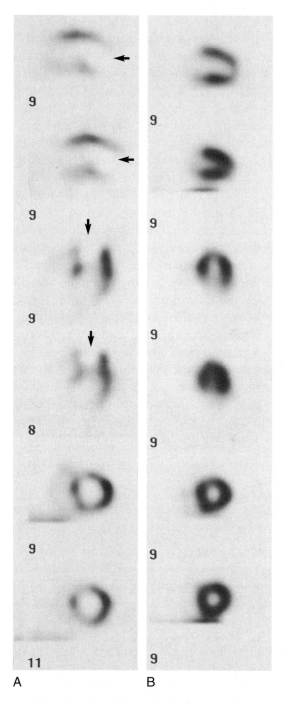

Figure 7-6. Myocardial stress/rest perfusion scan. (Left column) Images after exercise demonstrate a lack of isotope uptake (defect) in the apex of the heart (arrows). (Right column) At rest, this area shows normal isotope uptake (perfusion), indicating that the defect represents ischemia rather than infarction.

brought on by exercise (angina). They are also performed to visualize blood flow to the heart muscle (myocardial perfusion scan) (Fig. 7-6), demonstrate the extent of injury to the heart muscle after a heart attack (myocardial infarction), and assess the results of bypass surgery or other revascularization procedures designed to restore blood flow to the heart.

To evaluate the extent of suspected or known coronary artery disease, cardiac scans are often performed immediately after a patient has engaged in physical exercise (stress test), such as walking on a treadmill or pedaling a stationary bicycle for a few minutes. This maximizes blood flow throughout the heart and makes any blockages of the coronary arteries easier to detect. While exercising, blood pressure is measured at frequent intervals and the electrical activity of the heart is monitored on an electrocardiogram (ECG). You will be asked to exercise until one of the following occurs: you reach a heart rate specified for your age and physical condition; you are too tired to continue or short of breath; or you experience chest pain, leg pain, or other symptoms that make you to want to stop. When the blood flow to the heart has reached its peak, a radioactive tracer is injected intravenously. It circulates throughout the body and collects in the heart muscle. About 1 minute later, exercise is stopped and imaging begins. The post-stress images are then compared with the pictures taken at rest to determine if there are any areas of your heart that are receiving an insufficient amount of blood.

Patients who are unable to exercise are given a medicine that increases blood flow to the heart. This may cause a brief period of dizziness, nausea, shortness of breath, anxiety, and even mild chest pain. If these symptoms do not resolve rapidly, another drug can be given to stop the effects of the first medicine.

You should not consume or use alcohol, caffeine, or tobacco (or any other source of nicotine) for 24 hours before the test, since this could affect the results. Each cardiac scan takes about 15–30 minutes to perform, and the total time in the nuclear medicine department typically ranges from 2–4 hours.

Positron Emission Tomography (PET)

What Is PET?

Positron emission tomography (PET) is a nuclear medicine procedure that produces three-dimensional images of functional processes in the body. Positron emission tomography/computed tomography (PET/CT) is a hybrid imaging modality based on the mechanical fusion of PET and CT systems in the same scanner. For most uses, PET/CT has replaced PET alone, since it combines the exquisite anatomic detail of CT with the functional capabilities of PET to detect areas of abnormal metabolic activity (Fig. 7-7).

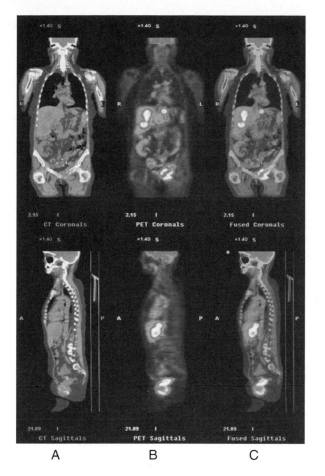

Figure 7-7. PET/CT of the body. (A) CT scan provides anatomic landmarks in the coronal (top) and sagittal (bottom) planes. (B) PET images show increased uptake, indicating a malignant tumor. (C) Combined PET/CT image provides greater detail by clearly localizing the anatomic position of the area of increased uptake.

This combination permits more accurate diagnosis than the two scans performed separately and actually decreases the duration of the procedure. In the future, PET also will be combined with MRI.

Why Am I Having this Test?

Positron emission tomography scanning is used to detect cancer, determine whether it has spread (metastasized), evaluate the response to therapy, and assess for recurrence; to study blood flow to the brain and the metabolic activity within it; and to assess blood flow to the heart muscle and detect areas damaged from a heart attack. Your physician may order a PET scan to evaluate:

- Cancer or lymphoma: early detection and determination of whether a mass is malignant or benign; to search for metastatic spread (when CT or MRI findings are inconclusive); to evaluate the response to treatment (decreased metabolic activity may be detected before anatomic changes are seen on CT or MRI) (Fig. 7-8); and to identify recurrence (PET is the most accurate technique for differentiating tumor recurrence from postsurgical change or radiation necrosis)
- Central nervous system disease (Fig. 7-9): differentiating Alzheimer's disease from other forms of dementia (such as Parkinson's disease, Huntington's disease, or vascular dementia); in patients with epilepsy, it is highly accurate in localizing areas of the brain causing seizures and determining whether surgery might be effective
- Coronary artery disease or heart attack: shows areas of decreased blood flow to the heart; identifies areas of heart muscle with inadequate blood flow that may benefit from a surgical procedure (bypass graft) or interventional radiology (angioplasty)

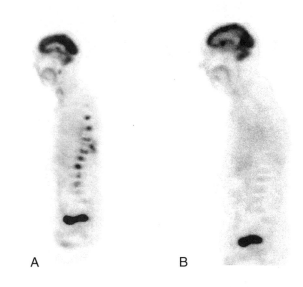

A   B

Figure 7-8. PET scan to assess effectiveness of chemotherapy. (A) Image before therapy shows multiple areas of abnormal radionuclide uptake. (B). After chemotherapy, there is substantially decreased uptake, indicating successful treatment.

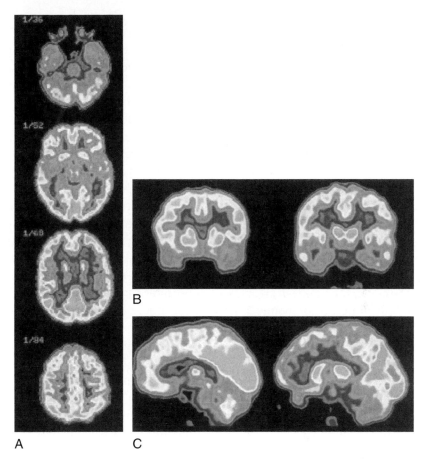

A   C

Figure 7-9. Normal PET images of the brain. (A) Axial or transverse, (B) coronal, and (C) sagittal images.

What Should I Tell My Doctor?

Before going for a radionuclide scan, make certain to tell your doctor if you:

- Are or might be pregnant
- Are breast feeding (if so, use formula and discard your breast milk for 1–2 days after the scan until the radioactive tracer has been eliminated from your body)

Why Was PET Scanning Developed and How Does It Work?

Plain radiographs, as well as more sophisticated techniques such as CT and MRI, may detect an abnormality but be unable to demonstrate whether it is benign or malignant. In the past, the patient often had to undergo biopsy, surgery, or an invasive imaging procedure to make this determination.

In PET scanning, the radionuclide (tracer) injected into your body is a biologically active molecule. The most frequently used tracer is a radio-active form of fluorine that is attached to a modified sugar (fluorodeoxy-glucose). Known as *18-FDG*, this tracer becomes concentrated in various tissues of the body in amounts directly related to their metabolic activity. The positrons (tiny positively charged particles) emitted by the radionuclide collide with tiny negatively charged particles (electrons), creating two high-energy gamma rays that are detected by the PET scanner. A sophisticated computer then transforms this information into images that can be viewed on a television-like monitor. Regions of increased metabolic activity and high tracer uptake appear as areas of high intensity (hot spots), whereas those with little or no chemical activity and tracer concentration produce areas of low intensity (cold spots).

One major purpose of PET scanning is to determine whether a nodule in the lung is benign or malignant. Cancer cells have higher metabolic rates than normal cells, so they show up as areas of high intensity on a PET scan. By highlighting areas with increased, decreased, or no metabolic activity, PET scanning can demonstrate areas in the brain causing epileptic seizures, help distinguish Alzheimer's disease from other causes of dementia, and determine the viability of heart muscle after a myocardial infarction and the potential success of revascularization procedures.

Positron emission tomography scans do not demonstrate as much detail as CT or MR images because they only show the location of the tracer. Therefore, most PET scanners today are combined with CT to provide excellent images demonstrating the precise anatomic areas of abnormal accumulation of the radionuclide tracer (Fig. 7-10). In the future, PET/MRI will add a third dimension to the test by providing additional metabolic information.

How Do I Prepare for a PET Scan?

There is no special preparation for a PET scan. You usually will be asked not to eat or drink fluids other than water for several hours before the exam-ination, since oral intake might alter the distribution of the radionuclide tracer in you body and cause a suboptimal scan that might have to be repeated on another day. If you are diabetic, your physician will give you

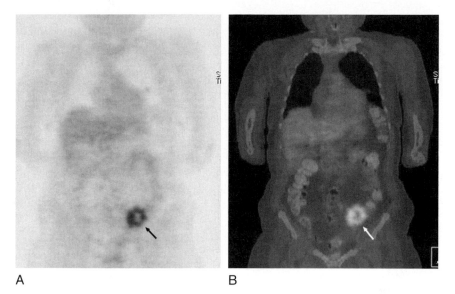

A   B

Figure 7-10. PET/CT scan of the body. (A) Initial PET scan shows an abnormal area of high metabolic area (arrow), but not enough anatomic detail to precisely localize it. (B) On the combined PET/CT scan, the excellent display of anatomy indicates that the hot area (arrow) represents an unexpected carcinoma of the sigmoid carcinoma.

special instructions to decrease the possibility of false results related to altered blood sugar or blood insulin levels.

What Does the Equipment Look Like?

A PET scanner is a large doughnut-shaped machine with a hole in the middle, similar in appearance to a CT or MRI unit (Fig. 7-11). Within the ring is a rotating array of detectors that captures the gamma rays (high-energy x-rays) given off by the process started with the injected radionuclide. The PET/CT scanner has all the components of both of these modalities mounted in the same gantry. A sophisticated computer system, often located in an adjacent room, processes all of the information about metabolic activity and transforms it into an image that can be seen on a television-like monitor.

How Is the Test Performed?

A PET scan is performed either in a hospital nuclear medicine department or in a special PET center. Depending on the area being examined, you may be asked to remove all or most of your clothes (you may be able to keep on your underwear) and be given a lightweight gown to wear. Your will be

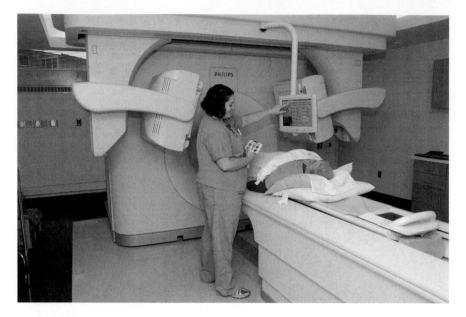

Figure 7-11. PET-CT scanner.

asked to lie on a bed or table, and the radioactive tracer will be injected into a vein in your arm. For a PET scan of the heart, electrodes for an ECG will be placed on your body. You may undergo two scans, one before and one after exercising. For a PET scan of the head, you may be asked to read, name letters, or tell a story, depending on whether the test is designed to evaluate your speech, reasoning, or memory.

During the scan, you must stay very still to get the highest-quality pictures and avoid blurring the images. After the procedure, you may be asked to wait for a few minutes until the technologist checks the images to make certain that no additional scanning is needed. Then you are free to leave the radiology facility and resume your normal activities. You will be instructed to drink a large amount of fluid and empty your bladder frequently for 1–2 days after the procedure to help flush the tracer from your body. It is important to remember that you do not pose a hazard to other people, since the tracer emits less radiation that a standard x-ray ray study.

A PET scan takes approximately 30 minutes, depending upon the body part being imaged and the instrument model

What Will I Feel?

A PET scan is completely painless. You will feel a slight pinprick as the intravenous needle goes through your skin. When the radionuclide is injected, you will not feel any different. For most people, the most difficult part of the test is lying on the back without moving while the scan is being made. A PET/CT scan actually takes less time than a PET scan alone, since the CT component is able to correct information from the PET component in less time than the previous non-CT method. Ask the technologist for a pillow or blanket to make yourself as comfortable as possible before the scanning begins.

What Are the Advantages and Disadvantages of PET Scanning?

Advantages

- Provides unique information regarding metabolic activity that cannot be obtained by other imaging techniques
- Noninvasive way to determine whether an abnormal area (detected on plain radiographs, CT, or MRI) is benign or malignant
- Permits scanning of the entire body on a single examination (valuable when searching for metastatic spread of tumor or a recurrence of disease after treatment)
- When combined with CT, PET provides a high level of anatomic accuracy in a single procedure; in the future, MRI will add functional and anatomic information to the metabolic information from PET
- Allergic reactions to the radioactive tracer are rare

Disadvantages

- More expensive than cross-sectional studies such as CT and MRI
- Poor spatial resolution of anatomic structures compared to other imaging techniques (but this problem is solved when PET is combined with CT or MRI)
- May give false results in patients with abnormal chemical balance (especially diabetics or patients who have eaten within a few hours prior to the examination)

8

ANGIOGRAPHY

Catheter Angiography

What Is Catheter Angiography?

Catheter angiography is an invasive x-ray test in which contrast material is injected through a thin plastic tube (catheter) inserted in the groin or arm to produce images of arteries and veins in various parts of the body. This procedure may be used to diagnose an arterial or venous abnormality and abnormal blood flow to a tumor. It also can be employed as an interventional technique to open up blocked blood vessels (angioplasty) and stop the hemorrhage from a vessel that is bleeding (embolization) without the need for surgery. The most common types of catheter angiography focus on the arteries to the heart, brain, and lower extremities.

In recent years, the use of catheter angiography for diagnostic purposes (except for coronary angiography) (Fig. 8-1) has been almost completely eliminated with the development of minimally invasive computed tomography angiography (CTA) and magnetic resonance angiography (MRA).

Why Am I Having this Test?

Catheter angiography is used to demonstrate abnormalities of the arteries and veins. Your physician may order this test as a diagnostic procedure if your clinical symptoms suggest:

- Atherosclerotic narrowing of an artery in the neck leading to the brain that could result in a stroke (carotid arteriogram), an artery supplying the heart that could cause a heart attack (coronary arteriogram), an artery leading to the kidney that may be causing high blood pressure (Fig. 8-2), or an artery to the leg causing pain on walking (aortogram or peripheral arteriogram)

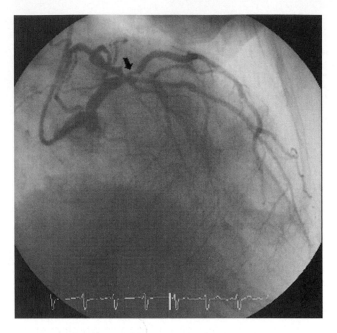

Figure 8-1. Coronary angiography. The arrow points to an area of atherosclerotic narrowing of the diagonal branch of the left main coronary artery.

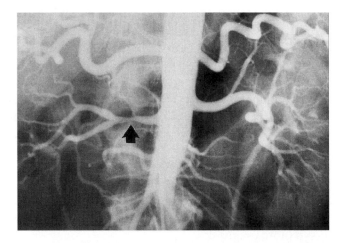

Figure 8-2. Renovascular hypertension. Arteriogram demonstrates narrowing of the right renal artery (arrow) causing the elevated blood pressure.

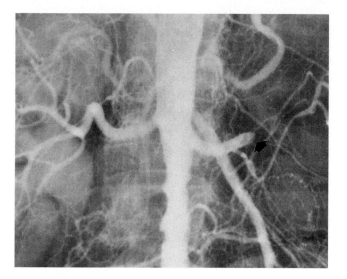

Figure 8-3. Acute embolic occlusion of the left renal artery. There is abrupt termination of the contrast column (arrow). The irregular contour of the aorta below the renal arteries represents diffuse atherosclerotic disease.

- Blockage of an artery due to clot (Fig. 8-3)
- An aneurysm (focal dilatation of an artery, due to a weakness in the wall, which could rupture and cause severe bleeding) (Fig. 8-4)
- Arterial rupture (tear in a blood vessel causing hemorrhage) or dissection (bleeding within the wall of an artery that can cause narrowing or even complete blockage) (Fig. 8-5)

Interventional catheter angiography (see p. 190) may be recommended to:

- Dilate a narrowed artery (angioplasty)
- Stop bleeding from a blood vessel (embolization)
- Decrease the blood supply to a vascular tumor to make it easier to remove it at surgery
- Place a stent across a diseased artery or vein to allow continued flow of blood through it

What Should I Tell My Doctor?

Before going for catheter angiography, make certain to tell your doctor if you:

- Are or suspect that you might be pregnant
- Are breast feeding (you may be able to pump breast milk ahead of time and use it for the first 24 hours after the angiogram; otherwise, throw

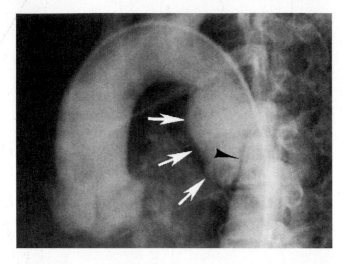

Figure 8-4. Pseudoaneurysm. Following trauma, an aortogram demonstrates an area of focal dilatation at the level of the aortic isthmus (arrows). The arrowhead points to the characteristic intimal flap.

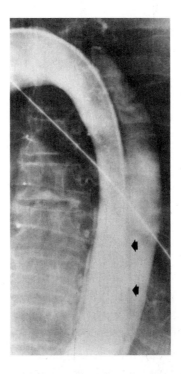

Figure 8-5. Aortic dissection. Aortogram demonstrates a thin radiolucent (dark) intimal flap separating the true and false aortic channels.

out your breast milk and use formula for 1–2 days after angiography until all the contrast material has been eliminated from your body)
- Are allergic to the iodinated contrast material used in the test
- Have ever had a serious allergic reaction (anaphylaxis) to any substance, such as a bee sting or eating shellfish
- Have asthma
- Have a history of kidney problems or diabetes, especially if you take metformin (Glucophage), since the contrast material used during angiography can damage the kidneys in those who have poor kidney function
- Are taking aspirin or another blood-thinning medicine

Why Was Catheter Angiography Developed and How Does It Work?

Arteries and veins cannot be demonstrated on plain radiographs. They require the use of iodinated contrast material, which makes them appear bright white on x-ray images. The radiologist places a catheter through the skin into an artery in your groin or arm and maneuvers it under the fluoroscope to position it as close as possible to the area of the body to be examined before injecting the contrast material and taking a series of images. For interventional procedures, a special catheter is used to dilate areas of narrowing (stenoses), while coils and various other materials can be introduced through a catheter to stop bleeding or clot off an aneurysm.

Historical vignette

Initially, angiographic studies were performed by injecting contrast material through a needle that was placed by a surgical procedure into the artery leading to the part of the body of clinical concern. Later, the needle was inserted by a direct puncture through the skin overlying an artery. The revolutionary development that paved the way for modern arteriography was the Seldinger technique. After the puncture of an artery in the groin or arm, a wire is inserted through the needle in the artery. Then the needle is withdrawn, a thin plastic tube (catheter) the same size as the needle (to prevent bleeding) is pushed over the wire, and the wire is removed, leaving only the catheter in place. The catheter can then be manipulated under fluoroscopic guidance so that it delivers the contrast material close to the area of interest. For example, when an arteriogram of the brain is performed, a catheter placed in an artery in the groin can be advanced into the carotid artery, thus avoiding the danger of directly puncturing this major blood vessel in the neck.

How Do I Prepare for Catheter Angiography?

Before any type of catheter angiography, your physician or the radiologist will describe how the procedure is performed, the meaning of various results, possible complications, and any alternative examinations so that you can sign an informed consent form (see p. 212). You may be asked to have tests of your kidney function (blood urea nitrogen, or BUN, and creatinine) and blood clotting (coagulation) studies.

Do not eat or drink anything for 4–8 hours before the angiogram. You may be asked not to take aspirin or other blood thinners for several days before the test and for 1 day after it.

What Does the Equipment Look Like?

The equipment used for catheter angiography typically consists of a radiographic table and a fluoroscopic unit with a television-like monitor that is located either in the examining room or nearby (Fig. 8-6). When the radiologist needs to view the fluoroscopic images in real time, the image intensifier (which converts x-rays into a video image) is positioned over the table on which you are lying. When the unit is used for taking still pictures, the image is captured either electronically or on film.

The catheter used in angiography is a long plastic tube that is about as thick as a strand of spaghetti. It is preshaped so that it tends to pass

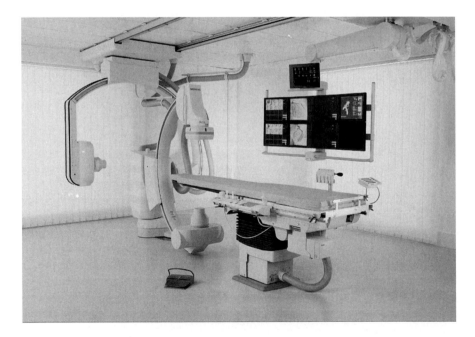

Figure 8-6. Cardiac catheterization equipment.

into the precise artery that may be abnormal or leads to the organ under investigation.

How Is the Test Performed?

You will be asked to remove some or all of your clothing (other than underwear) and be given a lightweight gown to wear during the examination. An IV line will be inserted into a small vein in your hand or arm before the procedure begins, just in case there is a need (infrequent) to give you medication or blood products during the study. A pulse oximeter, which measures the oxygen level in the blood, may be clipped to you finger or ear. Small discs (electrodes) may be placed on your arms, chest, or legs to record your heart rate and rhythm. A lead apron may be placed under your genital and pelvic areas to protect them from x-ray exposure (the x-ray source is within the table). You may be given a small dose of a sedative to keep you relaxed during the procedure.

The area of your groin or armpit where the catheter is to be inserted will be shaved, cleaned with an antiseptic agent, and numbed with a local anesthetic. The radiologist will make a small incision in the skin to make it easier for the needle to pass into the artery. When the stylet is removed from the needle, some blood usually spurts out until a long guidewire can be inserted into the needle. Once the guidewire is clearly within the artery, the needle is withdrawn and a catheter is slid over the length of the guidewire. The radiologist manipulates the catheter and guidewire under fluoroscopic guidance until it reaches the area to be studied. The guidewire is then removed, and the catheter is left in place in preparation for the administration of contrast material. This is injected either by hand with a syringe or mechanically by an automatic pressure injector attached to the catheter. The latter technique is commonly used because it can propel a large volume of contrast quickly. This provides a better image since there is less dilution of the contrast material by unopacified blood. During and for several seconds after the contract injection, a series of x-ray pictures are taken in rapid succession (because the contrast material passes swiftly through the area). While the images are being obtained, you will be asked to lie very still to prevent any blurring, and you may be asked to hold your breath for several seconds. To view the area of interest from different angles or perspectives, you may be asked to change positions for additional contrast injections.

Once the radiologist is satisfied that all of the required images have been obtained, the catheter is slowly and carefully removed. The IV line is also taken out. The incision site is closed by applying direct pressure on the puncture site for about 15 minutes or by using a closure device that seals the small hole made in the artery at the puncture site.

Catheter angiography may be completed in less than 1 hour, though complicated procedures may last for several hours. Therefore, you should empty your bladder just before the test begins.

What Postprocedure Care Will I Receive?

If you have catheter angiography as an outpatient, you will rest in bed in a recovery room for observation for 6–12 hours before you go home. (You may resume your normal diet immediately.) Rather than have you leave late in the evening, you may be admitted to the hospital overnight, especially if you live relatively far away. A nurse will periodically take your vital signs (blood pressure, pulse rate), check the peripheral pulses in the arm or leg where the catheter was inserted, and carefully observe the arterial puncture site to make certain that there is no bleeding. You may want to bring something to do or read to pass the time. Arrange to have someone take you home, because you may be given a sedative before the test. If you are given a sedative, do not drive for at least 24 hours.

If the catheter was placed in the groin area (femoral artery), you will be asked to keep that leg straight for several hours. You can use an ice pack on the needle puncture site to relieve any pain and swelling. Pain medication may be prescribed if needed. If the arterial puncture was performed in your armpit, you should not have any blood taken from that arm or have your blood pressure measured in that arm for several days.

Remember that it is normal for the puncture site to be sore and bruised for several weeks. An occasional complication after catheter angiography is the development of a hematoma, a hard mass caused by bleeding during the procedure. A hematoma should be watched carefully, since it may indicate continued bleeding of the arterial puncture site.

After catheter angiography, you may be advised to rest for 2–3 days to avoid placing any stress on the arterial puncture site. You should call your physician immediately if you experience:

- Continued bleeding or increasing swelling at the puncture site
- Numbness, tingling, pain, coolness, loss of color, or loss of function in the arm or leg where the catheter was inserted
- Sudden dizziness
- Chest pain or severe difficulty breathing
- Vision problems, slurred speech, or muscle weakness
- Any sign of infection (fever, chills, and red streaks or pus related to the puncture site)

What Will I Feel?

You will feel a pinprick when the IV line is inserted and may experience some stinging from the local anesthetic at the puncture site. There may be some pressure when the catheter is inserted through the skin, but you should not feel the catheter in your artery. If you experience any discomfort as the catheter is being positioned, let the radiologist know and you will be given some additional local anesthetic.

When the contrast material is injected, it is normal to feel warmth or a slight burning sensation. For some people the feeling of heat is strong, while for others it is mild. You may have flushing of the face and a salty or metallic taste in your mouth. Possible side effects or reactions include headache, dizziness, irregular heartbeat, nausea, and chest pain, but they usually last for only a few seconds. If you become light-headed or have difficulty breathing, notify the technologist immediately since this may indicate a more severe allergic reaction. In this infrequent occurrence, a radiologist or other physician is always available to provide immediate assistance. For most people, the most difficult part of the test is lying flat on the table for several hours. After the procedure, while you are in the recovery room, notify the nurse if you notice any bleeding, swelling, or pain at the puncture site where the catheter entered the skin.

What Are the Advantages and Disadvantages of Catheter Angiography Compared with CTA and MRA?

Advantages

- Ability to combine diagnosis and treatment in a single procedure (for example, if a narrowed artery is demonstrated, it may be dilated or a stent inserted)
- Interventional procedures may eliminate the need for surgery, or make surgery easier with less operative bleeding
- Provides the most detailed, clear, and accurate images of the blood vessels, especially if the catheter can be maneuvered close to the area of interest

Disadvantages

- Invasive procedure with risk of complications
- Uses a large amount of contrast material (not recommended for diabetics and individuals who have poor kidney function or are dehydrated)
- Dangerous in people with a previous reaction to contrast (though steroids can be given before the procedure if catheter angiography is essential)

- Risk of bleeding from the arterial puncture site is increased in patients who take blood thinners (anticoagulant medications)
- Carotid arteriography (of the neck) can lead to a stroke if a blood clot or plaque on the inside of the arterial wall is dislodged by the catheter and blocks a small artery to the brain
- Coronary arteriography (of the heart) can irritate the heart and produce arrhythmias (abnormal heartbeats)
- Involves more radiation exposure

CT Angiography (CTA)

What Is CTA?

Computed tomography angiography is a minimally invasive x-ray test in which contrast material injected intravenously permits detailed images of vascular structures throughout the body. In recent years, CTA (and MRA) have almost completely eliminated invasive catheter angiography for diagnostic purposes (except for coronary angiography).

Why Am I Having this Test?

Computed tomography angiography is used to demonstrate abnormalities of the arteries and veins, especially the presence and extent of atherosclerotic arterial disease. Your physician may order this test as a diagnostic procedure if your clinical symptoms suggest:

- Atherosclerotic narrowing of a neck artery leading to the brain that could result in a stroke (carotid angiogram), an artery supplying the heart that could cause a heart attack (coronary angiogram), or an artery to the leg (aortogram or peripheral arteriogram)
- An aneurysm (focal dilatation of an artery, due to a weakness in the wall, that could rupture and cause severe bleeding) (Fig. 8-7)
- Arterial rupture (tear in a blood vessel causing hemorrhage) or dissection (bleeding within the wall of an artery that can cause narrowing or even complete blockage)

In patients who have had previous arterial surgery or radiologic interventional procedures to dilate narrowed arteries, CTA is the ideal follow-up study to evaluate the patency of native arteries, bypass grafts, and stents and thus determine whether additional surgery or other interventional procedures are needed.

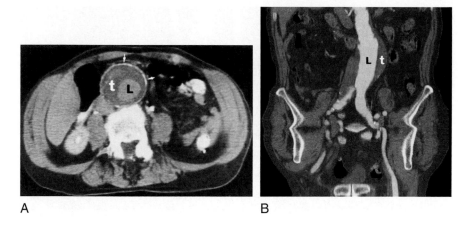

A   B

Figure 8-7. Abdominal aortic aneurysm. (A) Axial CT scan shows a low-density thrombus (t) surrounding the blood-filled lumen (L). The wall of the aneurysm contains high-density calcification (arrows). (B) Coronal reconstruction CTA shows an abdominal aortic aneurysm beginning below the renal arteries and extending below the iliac bifurcation.

What Should I Tell My Doctor?

Before going for CTA, make certain to tell your doctor if you:

- Are or suspect that you might be pregnant
- Are allergic to the iodinated contrast material used in the test
- Have ever had a serious allergic reaction (anaphylaxis) to any substance, such as a bee sting or eating shellfish
- Have asthma
- Have a history of kidney problems or diabetes, especially if you take metformin (Glucophage), since the contrast material used during angiography can damage the kidneys in those who have poor kidney function

Why Was CTA Developed and How Does It Work?

Arteries and veins cannot be demonstrated on plain radiographs and require the use of iodinated contrast material, which makes them appear bright white on x-ray images. Initially, this problem was solved using catheter angiography (see p. 163), in which the radiologist places a catheter through the skin into the arterial system and maneuvers it under fluoroscopic guidance as close as possible to the area of the body to be examined before injecting the contrast material and taking a series of images. However, this is an invasive and prolonged procedure associated with an appreciable complication rate. The development of multidetector CT scanners, which allow very thin slices to be obtained rapidly, permits detailed images of arteries

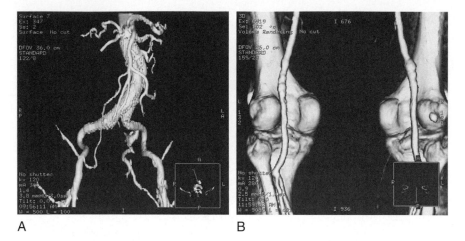

A   B

Figure 8-8. CT angiography. (A) Special software permits subtraction of overlying structures to visualize in exquisite detail the abdominal aorta, the renal arteries, the superior mesenteric artery, and the iliac arteries. (B) Three-dimensional (3D) image of the popliteal arteries around both knees.

and veins that are comparable to those of catheter angiography (Fig. 8-8) but noninvasively and with far fewer complications.

How Do I Prepare for a CTA Scan?

You should wear comfortable, loose-fitting clothing, though you may have to take off some of your clothes. You will be given a gown to put on during the procedure. Because metal objects such as eyeglasses, dentures, hairpins, and jewelry can produce artifacts that degrade the image, they may have to be removed, depending on the part of your body being examined.

You will be asked to fast (no solids or liquids) for 4–6 hours before the examination. This is done to prevent aspiration of stomach contents if you have a contrast reaction, which is fortunately uncommon.

Remember that the CT scanner has a weight limit to prevent damage to its internal mechanisms. If you weigh more than 350 pounds, it is possible that you may not be able to have the test performed.

What Does the Equipment Look Like?

A CT scanner consists of three parts, two of which you will see. The machine itself looks like a large doughnut, which contains the many x-ray tubes and electronic detectors located opposite each other in a ring called a *gantry*, which rotates around you. You will be placed on a movable examination table, which slides into and out of the hole in the doughnut. The third part of the CT scanner is the sophisticated computer that processes all of the imaging information; it is located in a separate room.

How Is the Test Performed?

A CTA is usually performed on an outpatient basis. You will be asked to lie on the narrow table that slides into the center of the scanner. In most cases you will be asked to lie on your back, though occasionally it is necessary to be on your front or side. Straps and pillows may be used to help you maintain the correct position and remain motionless during the examination.

A nurse or technologist will insert an IV into a small vein in your hand or arm. A small dose of contrast material may be injected through the IV to determine how long it takes to reach the area under study. For the actual CTA, an automatic injection machine connected to the IV will inject contrast material at a controlled rate both prior to and during scanning. The number of doses of contrast material and the precise timing vary, depending on the area of the body examined.

The first step is for the technologist to take a scout image to test the radiographic technique and to determine the correct starting position for the actual CT scan. For this brief part of the procedure, the table moves quickly through the scanner. Once the actual CT scan is being performed, the table moves more slowly through the machine. To prevent motion that blurs the image, the technician will inform you when to hold your breath and not move. Each set of images is obtained within 5–15 seconds. However, your actual time in the scanner will be longer (often up to 30 minutes) as the technologist positions you on the table, checks or places the IV line, performs the preliminary injection, and then enters the parameters for the injection and image acquisition sequence into the computer. After the procedure has been completed, you will be asked to wait for several minutes until the technologist determines that the study is of sufficiently high quality for the radiologist to read. The IV line will then be removed, and you can return to your normal activities.

What Will I Feel?

The x-rays in a CTA are painless. The main discomfort will probably be the need to lie still on the hard table. If the room is too cool, you can ask for a blanket. If you have chronic pain or are claustrophobic, tell the technologist and you may be able to receive medication to ease the pain or let you relax.

During the actual CT scan, there will be a slight metallic sound (buzzing, clicking, whirring) as the scanner revolves around you.

When the IV contrast material is given, you may feel a slight burning sensation in the arm in which it is injected, a metallic taste in the mouth, and a warm flushing of the body. These sensations are normal and usually subside within a few seconds. The most common complication of contrast material is itching and hives, which is relieved with medication. Some patients may feel nauseous. If you become light-headed or have difficulty breathing, notify the technologist immediately since this may indicate a more severe but rare allergic reaction. In the unlikely event of a contrast reaction, a radiologist or another physician is always available to provide immediate assistance.

Although you are alone in the CT room during the examination, the technologist will always be able to see you through the special leaded glass window and answer any questions through a two-way intercom. Parents may be permitted to remain in the examination room with children, though they will be required to wear a lead apron to prevent radiation exposure.

What Are the Advantages and Disadvantages of CTA Compared with Catheter Angiography?

Advantages

- Minimally invasive procedure with low risk of complications
- Rapid study with less radiation exposure

Disadvantages

- Catheter angiograph has the ability to combine diagnosis and treatment in a single procedure (for example, if a narrowed artery is demonstrated, it may be dilated or a stent inserted)

Special Types of CTA

CT Coronary Arteriography

Computed tomography coronary arteriography is a new, minimally invasive imaging test to diagnose diseases of the heart. Two of the most important applications are the detection of atherosclerotic coronary artery disease and the follow-up of patients who have undergone coronary bypass surgery. In the past, there were only two ways to assess the status of the coronary arteries. Noninvasive functional studies, such as treadmill tests and radionuclide examinations, provide indirect information about possible blockages in the coronary arteries. Heart catheterization can directly demonstrate the coronary arteries, but this is an invasive procedure with an appreciable complication rate.

Single-slice CT scanning could visualize the heart, but its rapid beating made it impossible to demonstrate the small coronary arteries. A new generation of multislice CT scanners permits such rapid acquisition of images that the coronary arteries can be routinely seen in great detail. The ability to reformat CT images in various planes now makes it possible to produce two-dimensional (Fig. 8-9) and computer-generated three-dimensional (Fig. 8-10) images of the coronary arteries that rival or surpass those provided by catheter coronary angiography.

A normal CT coronary arteriogram virtually eliminates the possibility of significant coronary artery disease. Therefore, currently the most important role of this test is to reliably exclude narrowing or blockage of the vessels supplying the heart in a minimally invasive way. Moreover, CT coronary arteriography can demonstrate atherosclerotic plaques in the walls of the coronary arteries, as well as arterial narrowing that decreases blood flow and may cause symptoms of chest pain. If a substantial area of narrowing is detected, you may be a candidate for surgery or for an interventional radiologic procedure that can prevent the disease from progressing to complete blockage of a coronary artery that results in a heart attack.

Should Everyone Have CT Coronary Arteriography?

Computed tomography coronary arteriography should *not* be used as a screening test for coronary artery disease in the general population. At this

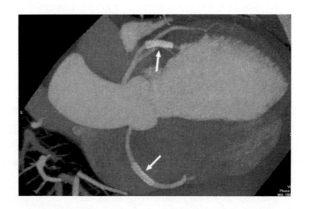

Figure 8-9. CT coronary arteriography. CT scan demonstrates metallic stents (arrows) that permit normal blood flow through previously narrowed coronary arteries.

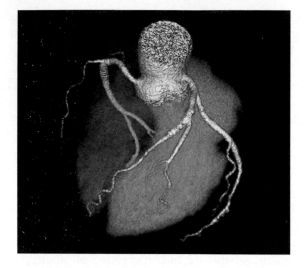

Figure 8-10. CT coronary arteriography. Three-dimensional CT image shows the coronary arteries in relation to the ventricles of the heart (in the background).

time, the use of CT coronary arteriography is considered most helpful in individuals who have atypical symptoms or unclear stress-test results. A normal or only mildly abnormal CT scan excludes severe coronary artery disease. Conversely, a significantly abnormal CT coronary arteriogram is an indication for either coronary artery bypass grafting or an interventional radiologic procedure to dilate the narrowed coronary artery (angioplasty) or place a stent across the diseased portion.

Experts disagree as to whether CT coronary arteriography should be performed in individuals who do not have symptoms (such as chest pain) but are at high risk for developing coronary artery disease. Some argue that CT coronary arteriography should be considered in people with a strong family history of vascular disease (heart attack and stroke), heavy cigarette smokers, and people with hypertension, diabetes, and high cholesterol levels.

Most experts agree that CT coronary arteriography is not an adequate substitute for catheter angiography in individuals with strong clinical evidence of coronary artery narrowing. This includes people with a prior heart attack or a known history of coronary artery disease, positive stress-test results, or a history of chest pain related to heavy physical activity. Computed tomography coronary arteriography also is of limited value in elderly individuals with extensive old, calcified plaque. Individuals who are seriously overweight or have abnormal heart rhythms also may not be good candidates for CT coronary arteriography, because these conditions may cause significant blurring that decreases image quality.

The decision on whether to have CT coronary arteriography should be made in consultation with your primary care physician or cardiologist. Although this procedure is only minimally invasive, it does involve x-ray exposure and there is the possibility of a serious allergic reaction to the IV contrast material.

CT Pulmonary Arteriography

Computed tomography pulmonary arteriography is now generally accepted as the best imaging study to detect pulmonary embolism, a blockage of the pulmonary artery or one of its branches. This usually happens when a blood clot from a vein in the leg or pelvis (deep vein thrombosis, or DVT) breaks loose and travels (embolizes) to the arterial supply of one of the lungs. Pulmonary emboli most commonly occur in hospitalized patients, in women taking birth control pills, and in individuals whose limbs have been immobilized for an extended period (such as in a cast after bone fracture or during extended air travel). Typical symptoms include difficulty breathing, chest pain on inspiration, rapid breathing, and heart palpitations. In severe cases, pulmonary embolism can lead to respiratory collapse, instability of the cardiovascular system, and sudden death.

Pulmonary embolism can be difficult to diagnose, especially in persons with underlying heart or lung disease. Plain chest radiographs are normal in more than half of the cases. Even when they are abnormal, the findings are nonspecific. In the past, the diagnostic study of choice was the radionuclide lung scan (see p. 148), also known as a *ventilation-perfusion scan* (*V/Q scan*). In this procedure, a small amount of radioactive tracer (radioisotope) is inhaled to study the flow of air to the lungs (ventilation), while a small amount of a different radioisotope is injected through an IV line to assess pulmonary blood flow (perfusion). Images are made of both studies and compared to detect indirectly the areas of lung affected by a pulmonary embolism. However, this examination is often difficult to obtain outside of normal working hours and is associated with a large number of indeterminate results that require further imaging studies.

In the past, the gold standard for demonstrating a pulmonary embolus was catheter pulmonary arteriography, which provides a detailed picture of blood flow to the lung. However, this test is time-consuming and technically difficult to perform. It is also associated with a significant rate of serious complications, including death.

In most radiology facilities today, CT pulmonary arteriography has replaced radionuclide lung scanning for making the diagnosis of pulmonary

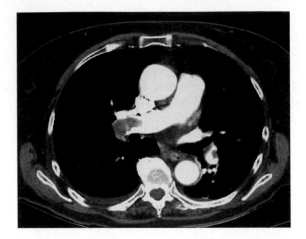

Figure 8-11. Pulmonary embolism. CT scan demonstrates a filling defect of the right pulmonary artery.

embolism. This technique is much faster and is readily available. Rather than indirectly suggesting the presence of a pulmonary embolism, CT pulmonary arteriography can demonstrate the embolism itself as a filling defect (dark) within an opaque (white) pulmonary artery (Fig. 8-11).

Magnetric Resonance Angiography (MRA)

What Is MRA?

Magnetic resonance angiography is a noninvasive test that uses a powerful magnetic field and pulses of radio wave energy to obtain detailed pictures of vascular structures throughout the body. In recent years, MRA (and CTA) have almost completely replaced invasive catheter angiography for diagnostic purposes (except for coronary angiography).

Why Am I Having this Test?

Magnetic resonance angiography is used to demonstrate diseases and anomalies of the arteries and veins, especially the presence and extent of atherosclerotic arterial disease (Fig. 8-12). Your physician may order this test as a diagnostic procedure if your clinical symptoms suggest:

- Atherosclerotic narrowing of a neck artery leading to the brain that could result in a stroke (carotid arteriogram), an artery to the leg

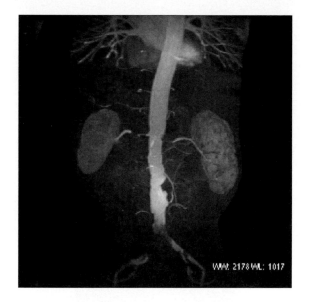

Figure 8-12. Atherosclerotic disease of the abdominal aorta and its branches. MRA shows irregular narrowing of the lower aorta and the iliac arteries.

(aortogram or peripheral arteriogram), or an artery to any organ that might cause it to malfunction
- An aneurysm (focal dilatation of an artery, due to a weakness in the wall, that could rupture and cause severe bleeding) (Figs. 8-13, 8-14)
- Arterial rupture (tear in a blood vessel causing hemorrhage) or dissection (bleeding within the wall of an artery that can cause narrowing or even complete blockage)

What Should I Tell My Doctor?

Before going for an MRA, make certain to tell your doctor if you:

- Are or might be pregnant or are breast feeding
- Are allergic to any medicine (unlike with CTA, the contrast material used for MRI does not contain iodine)
- Have kidney disease that may prevent you from being given gadolinium, the most commonly used MRA contrast material
- Have any of the metallic devices listed under MRI (see p. 102)
- Become nervous when in small spaces (claustrophobia); if so, you may need a sedative to relax and keep still (you should arrange for someone to take you home after the procedure); note that this is less of a problem with open magnets

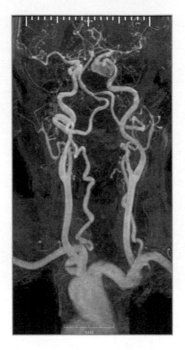

Figure 8-13. MRA of an aneurysm of the cavernous portion of the left internal carotid artery.

- Are unable to lie on your back for 30–60 minutes
- Weigh more than 300 pounds

Why Was MRA Developed and How Does It Work?

Arteries and veins cannot be demonstrated on plain radiographs and require the use of iodinated contrast material, which makes them appear bright white on x-ray images. Initially, this problem was solved using catheter angiography (see p. 163), in which the radiologist places a catheter through the skin into the arterial system and maneuvers it under fluoroscopic guidance as close as possible to the area of the body to be examined before injecting the contrast material and taking a series of images. However, this is an invasive and prolonged procedure associated with an appreciable complication rate. The development of thin-slice MRI scanners permits detailed images of arteries and veins that in some areas of the body are comparable to those of catheter angiography but noninvasively and with far fewer complications.

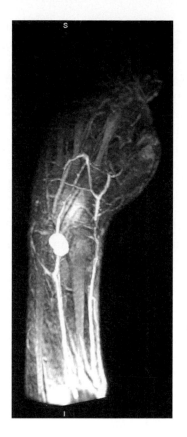

Figure 8-14. MRA of a pseudoaneurysm of the ulnar artery in the wrist.

How Do I Prepare for MRA?

The key to preparation for MRA is to remember that *no* metal objects are allowed in the examination room and should be left at home if possible. In rare cases, a large metallic object can cause severe injury if it flies through the air at great speed toward the magnet. Objects that should not be taken into the room with the magnet include:

- Jewelry, watches, credit cards with magnetic strips, and hearing aids (can be damaged by the strong magnetic field)
- Pins, hairpins, and metal zippers (can distort the images)
- Removable dentures
- Eyeglasses, pens, and pocket knives
- Body piercings

If you bring any metal objects with you, they must be removed before the MRA scan and placed in a secured locker that is available to store personal possessions.

In general, MRA is safe for patients with most metal implants (such as heart valves), though you should always make certain that your physician is aware of them before ordering the study You also should mention them to the technologist (or radiologist) before entering the MR scanning area. However, if you have the following implants, you should *not* go into the room where the MR examination is performed unless explicitly instructed to do so by a radiologist or technologist who is aware that you have one of them:

- Internal (implanted) heart pacemaker or defibrillator
- Implanted infusion pump (such as an insulin pump for diabetes, a narcotics pump for pain medication, or a nerve stimulator for back pain)
- Cochlear (ear) implant
- Some types of surgical clips used to clamp off brain aneurysms

In general, metal objects used in orthopedic surgery (pins, screws, plates, or surgical staples) pose no risk during MRA. However, a recently placed artificial joint (hip, knee) may require the use of another imaging procedure. If there is any question, an x-ray image can be obtained to determine whether you have a metallic object in your body. Similarly, a preliminary x-ray may be needed if you have a tattoo (some contain iron and could heat up during an MRA) or a history of an accident or working near metal that could have resulted in some tiny fragments lodged around your eye.

What Does the Equipment Look Like?

Magnetic resonance imaging scanners consist of three parts, two of which you will see. The machine itself is a large cylindrical tube that looks somewhat like a huge doughnut and contains the magnet and detectors. You will be placed on a movable examination table that slides in and out of the center of the magnet. The third part of the scanner is the sophisticated computer that processes all of the imaging information; it is located in a separate room.

There are two other major magnet configurations. *Short-bore* systems are designed so that you are not completely surrounded by the magnet; *open* magnets are open on all sides. These units are especially helpful for examining claustrophobic patients who are fearful of being in a closed space and for those who are very obese and do not fit in the standard MRI scanner.

How Is the Test Performed?

When you arrive at the radiology imaging facility, you may be asked to remove some or all of your clothing (especially anything with metal fasteners) and change into a lightweight gown to wear during the examination. If you are allowed to keep some of your clothes on, you will be asked to empty your pockets of all coins and cards with scanner strips (such as ATM and credit cards), since the MRI magnet may erase the information on them.

You will be asked to lie down on the movable examination table that slides into the middle of the magnet. Bolsters and straps may be used to support you and help maintain the proper position during the study. If you are extremely anxious when placed inside the MRI magnet, you may be given a sedative to make you more relaxed so that you can remain motionless.

Small devices that contain coils capable of sending and receiving radio waves may be placed around or adjacent to the area of the body to be scanned. A special belt strap may be used to sense your breathing or heartbeat, triggering the machine to take the images at the proper time.

If contrast material will be used in your MRA exam, a nurse or technologist will insert an IV line into a vein in your hand or arm. A saline solution will drip through the IV to keep the line open until the contrast material is injected after the initial series of scans. Additional images will be taken following the injection.

When the MR images are being obtained, you will hear loud, repetitive clicking and humming noises that may sound like machine gun fire. You may be given ear plugs or headphones with music to reduce the noise. Magnetic resonance imaging examinations generally include multiple runs (sequences), some of which may take several minutes to perform. During this time, it is critical that you lie completely still and breathe normally to prevent blurring of the images. At times, you may be asked to hold your breath for short periods of time.

The technologist will leave the MRI room and go to the control room while the examination is being performed. However, the technologist will always be able to see you through the control-room window and will be in voice contact with you via a two-way intercom system throughout the test. Some facilities permit a parent or friend to stay in the room.

The scanning time for an MRI examination depends on the area of the body studied and the number of sequences required. It usually takes about 30–60 minutes but can last as long as 2 hours. When the examination is completed, you may be asked to wait until the technologist checks the images, just in case additional sequences are needed. If you have received IV contrast material, the line will be removed. There is no recovery period after an MRI examination. Once the study is over, you are free to leave the radiology facility and resume your normal diet and activities.

What Will I Feel?

Most MRI examinations are painless, and you will not feel any effect from the magnetic field or the radio waves. You may find it uncomfortable to remain still during the procedure or experience a sense of being closed in (claustrophobia). Remember that sedation can be arranged if you think you will be extremely anxious, but fewer than 1 in 20 patients actually requires it. If you have metal dental fillings, you may feel a tingling sensation in your mouth.

You will always know when images are being obtained because you will hear the loud tapping or thumping sounds when the coils generate the radiofrequency pulses. Each sequence may take a few seconds or a few minutes. You will be able to relax between the imaging sequences, but you should maintain your position as much as possible. After the procedure is over, you may feel tired or sore from lying in one position for a long time on the hard table. The room may feel cool because of the air conditioning needed to protect the sensitive machinery.

For some types of MRA examinations, you will be asked to hold your breath for a few seconds. Remember that it is normal for the area of your body being imaged to feel slightly warm. If it feels very hot, notify the technologist. If you receive contrast material, it is normal to feel coolness and flushing for a minute or two. A few patients experience nausea and an allergic reaction of hives or itchy eyes. The IV needle may cause some discomfort when it is inserted, and you may feel some bruising when it is removed.

It is recommended that nursing mothers not breast-feed for 24 hours after an MRI examination with contrast material.

What Are the Advantages and Disadvantages of MRA Compared with CTA?

Advantages

- No exposure to radiation (x-rays)
- No known harmful effects from the strong magnetic fields used
- Higher spatial and soft-tissue contrast resolution, along with possible dynamic scanning
- Ability to image directly in multiple planes without the need to reformat the images

- The contrast used in MRA (gadolinium) is less likely to cause an allergic reaction than the iodine-based materials used for CT scanning and catheter angiography (though it can be dangerous in patients with pre-existing kidney disease)
- May be used in pregnant women since, unlike CTA, it involves no ionizing radiation. Although there is no reason to believe that MRI harms the fetus, pregnant women usually are advised not to have this study unless it is medically necessary

Disadvantages

- Longer, more expensive procedure
- The powerful magnet used in MRA prevents it from being used if you have an internal (implanted) heart pacemaker or defibrillator; an implanted infusion pump (such as an insulin pump for diabetes, a narcotics pump for pain medication, or a nerve stimulator for back pain); a cochlear (ear) implant; some types of surgical clips used to clamp off brain aneurysms; or metal fragments near the eye (a preliminary plain radiograph may be required to exclude this possibility)
- The powerful magnet may stop a nearby watch; erase information on ATM and credit cards; pull any loose metal objects toward it (possibly causing injury); or cause iron pigments in tattoos or tattooed eyeliner to produce skin or eye irritation or a burn from some medication patches
- In persons with poor kidney function, high doses of MRI contrast material have been associated with a very rare but possibly serious condition called *nephrogenic systemic sclerosis*
- Claustrophobia from the need to lie for a prolonged period in a closed area inside the magnetic tube
- Loud noise produced during the examination
- Requires patients to lie perfectly still for up to several minutes (CTA takes only a few seconds) or hold their breath for up to 30 seconds lest motion degrade the quality of the images
- Unlike CTA, MRA cannot image calcium deposits in atherosclerotic arterial plaques
- The sharpness of detail of MRA does not yet match that of CTA or catheter angiography, and at times it may be difficult to distinguish arteries from veins

9

INTERVENTIONAL RADIOLOGY

Many conditions that once required surgery can now be treated by interventional radiologists without the need for an operative procedure (Fig. 9-1). Among the many types of interventional procedures are:

- Dilatation of narrowed or blocked arteries to prevent heart attack and stroke (angioplasty)
- Embolization of arteries to stop bleeding or obstruct the blood supply to a tumor
- Ablation (destruction) of tumors without harming the normal healthy surrounding tissue.

Interventional procedures can be performed using fluoroscopy, ultrasound, CT, or MRI. The major advantages of interventional radiology include:

- Substantially less risk, pain, and recovery time
- Most procedures can be performed on an outpatient basis or require only a short stay in the hospital
- General anesthesia is usually not needed
- Often less expensive than surgery when the cost of hospitalization is considered

Before any type of interventional radiology procedure, your radiologist will describe how it is performed, the meaning of various results, possible complications, and any alternative examinations so that you can sign an informed consent form (see p. 212). You may be asked to have tests of your kidney function (blood urea nitrogen, or BUN, and creatinine) and blood clotting (coagulation) studies. Do not eat or drink anything for 4–8 hours

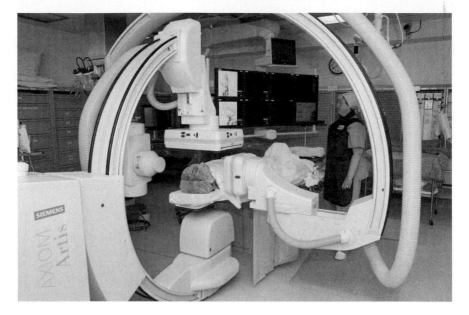

Figure 9-1. Interventional radiology room.

before the angiogram. You may be asked not to take aspirin or other blood thinners for several days before the test and for 1 day after it.

For convenience, interventional radiology procedures can be divided into two types—vascular (those involving blood vessels) and nonvascular.

Vascular Procedures

Percutaneous Transluminal Angioplasty (PTA)

Percutaneous transluminal angioplasty is a procedure to improve blood flow by opening up an artery that has been narrowed or blocked by fatty deposits of atherosclerotic disease. It is most commonly used in the following areas:

- Carotid artery (neck)—to increase blood flow to the brain and prevent a stroke
- Coronary artery—to increase blood flow to the heart, to treat ischemia, and to prevent a myocardial infarction (heart attack) (Fig. 9-2)
- Aorta and its branches
- Renal artery—to increase blood flow to the kidney and treat some forms of high blood pressure (hypertension) (Fig. 9-3)

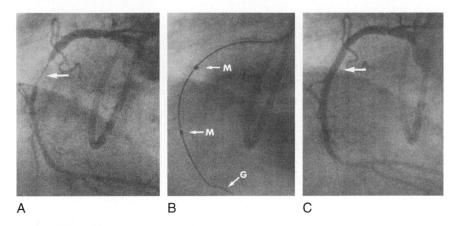

Figure 9-2. PTA for ischemia. (A) Initial angiogram shows severe narrowing (arrow) of the midportion of the right coronary artery. (B) During the PTA procedure, a steerable guide wire (G) is passed down the coronary artery and through the region of narrowing. Radiopaque markers (M) identify the balloon portion of the dilating catheter that has been advanced over the guide wire through the narrowed area. (C) Immediately after angioplasty, the previous site of narrowing (arrow) in now patent.

- Peripheral arteries (pelvis or leg)—to treat symptoms of claudication (pain in the lower extremity with exercise) (Fig. 9-4)
- Dialysis fistula or graft (placed in patients with kidney failure requiring dialysis)

During the procedure, a long, thin, flexible plastic tube (catheter) with a balloon at its end is inserted into an artery in your groin or arm. When the catheter has been advanced under fluoroscopy into the narrowed or blocked area, the balloon is slowly inflated and deflated several times (for about 20–60 seconds each time) with a pump that is filled with contrast material so that the radiologist can see changes in the size of the balloon in the artery on a television-like monitor. As the balloon inflates, it pushes the fatty deposits against the arterial wall. When the artery has been opened and normal blood flow has been restored and documented on images, the balloon catheter is removed.

A small tube (sheath) attached to a monitoring system may be left in the artery for 2–4 hours after the procedure or overnight to make certain that the blood is flowing smoothly. At times, a small wire mesh tube (stent) is permanently placed in the newly opened artery to support its damaged wall and help it remain patent. Like catheters, stents come in various sizes to match the width of the disease artery.

The entire PTA procedure usually takes about 90 minutes. After the catheter or sheath is removed, a doctor or nurse will either apply pressure to the

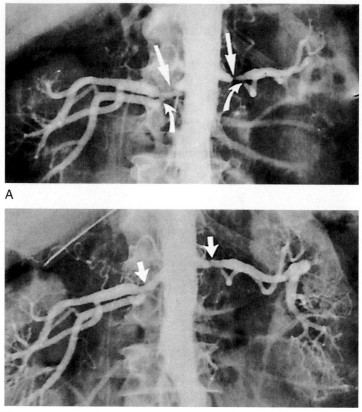

A

B

Figure 9-3. PTA for renovascular hypertension. (A) Abdominal aortogram demonstrates severe bilateral narrowing of the main renal arteries (straight arrows) and at the origins of early bifurcations of these vessels (curved arrows). (B) Repeat study after angioplasty of both renal arteries shows irregularities in areas of previous atherosclerotic narrowing (arrows), but an improved residual lumen in both main renal arteries. After the procedure, the patient's previous severe hypertension was controllable to normal levels with only minimal dosages of diuretic medication.

puncture site for about 15 minutes or use a closure device that seals the puncture site in the artery. For several hours, this area will be checked periodically for bleeding and your blood pressure and heart rate will be monitored. In most cases, you will be required to stay in bed for a few hours and will then be allowed to go home either the same day or the next. You may be asked to take a blood thinner (aspirin or prescription medicine) for a variable period to prevent blood clots from forming at the site of the angioplasty as the arterial wall heals. (For further information regarding what you will feel during the procedure, see the subsection "What Will I Feel?" in the section "Catheter Angiography" in Chapter 8, p. 171)

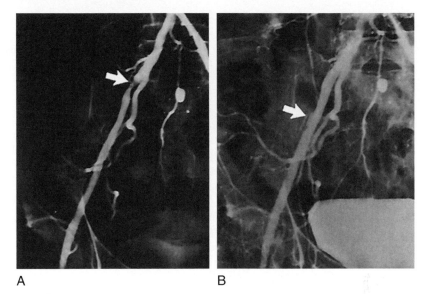

A   B

Figure 9-4. PTA for claudication. (A) Initial image shows narrowing of the right external iliac artery (arrow). (B) After angioplasty, there is relief of the narrowing (arrow). The patient's symptoms of pain in the leg with exercise completely disappeared.

Remember that PTA does not reverse or cure the underlying disease of atherosclerosis. To prevent recurrent arterial disease, it is extremely important that you quit smoking, eat a healthy diet that is low in saturated fat, and exercise regularly. If your have diabetes, high blood pressure, or high cholesterol, you need to follow rigorously the treatment plan prescribed by your doctor.

Embolization

Embolization is a procedure in which a medication or synthetic material is placed directly into an artery through a catheter to decrease blood flow. In many cases, this can prevent complicated and risky surgery. The most common uses of embolization include:

- Controlling or stopping bleeding (hemorrhage into the abdomen and pelvis after motor vehicle accidents or related to gastrointestinal tract disorders such as ulcers and diverticular disease) (Fig. 9-5)
- Treating an aneurysm (a bulge in a weak arterial wall), either by blocking the artery supplying blood to the aneurysm or by closing off the aneurysmal sac itself
- Occluding abnormal connections between arteries and veins (arteriovenous malformation or fistula)

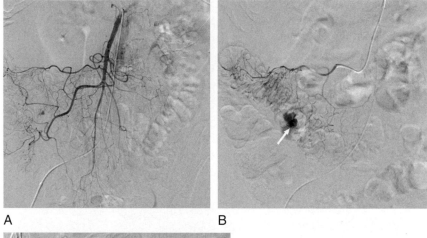

A   B

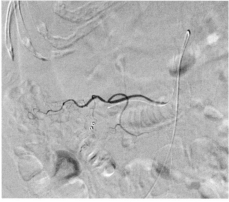

C

Figure 9-5. Embolization for upper GI bleeding. (Left) Contrast injection of the superior mesenteric artery shows a faint area of bleeding from a small branch to the right colon. (Middle) Selective catheterization of the right colic artery branch using a microcatheter. Contrast injection clearly shows the area of active arterial bleeding (arrow). (Right) Post-embolization contrast injection after small fibered platinum coils were deployed in the tiny feeding artery shows successful occlusion of the bleeding vessel.

- Blocking arteries supplying blood to a tumor that cannot be removed surgically or decreasing blood flow to a tumor so that it can be removed surgically with much less bleeding
- Providing palliative treatment of primary or metastatic liver cancer (see below)
- An alternative to hysterectomy (surgical removal of the uterus) in women with fibroid tumors causing long menstrual periods or heavy menstrual bleeding (uterine artery embolization; see below)

During the procedure, a long, thin, flexible plastic tube (catheter) is inserted into an artery in your groin or arm. When the catheter has been advanced under fluoroscopy into the artery leading to the bleeding site or tumor, the radiologist will select an appropriate embolization agent, depending on the size of the blood vessel or malformation and whether the treatment is designed to be temporary or permanent. Some of the most popular embolization agents are:

- Gelfoam—trade name for a gelatin sponge material that is cut into small pieces and floats downstream after being injected into an artery. This is a temporary measure because the material dissolves within several weeks.
- Particulate agents—gelatin-coated microspheres or polyvinyl alcohol (plastic material resembling coarse sand) suspended in liquid and injected into the bloodstream. These are intended to permanently block small vessels, including the treatment of bleeding fibroid tumors in the uterus.
- Coils—metallic devices made of stainless steel or platinum used to block large, fast-flowing arteries. They can be positioned precisely and are especially effective in stopping bleeding from an injured artery or blocking arterial blood flow into an aneurysm. A complication is the small risk of a coil being dislodged from the area where it was originally placed.
- Sclerosing agents—liquids such as alcohols that can destroy arteries and eliminate vessel malformations by causing blood clots to form within them
- Liquid glue—hardens quickly to rapidly close off a vessel

The embolization agent is introduced through a catheter that is positioned under fluoroscopy within the bleeding vessel or malformation, or into the artery supplying blood flow to a uterine fibroid or other tumor. Small amounts of contrast material are injected to make certain that the catheter is in the proper position. For arteriovenous malformations in the brain, test contrast injections are made to ensure that the artery into which the embolization agent is to be introduced does not supply any critical area. To completely treat a large arteriovenous malformation, multiple embolization procedures may be required on separate days.

Depending on the complexity of the underlying condition, an embolization procedure can take 30 minutes to several hours to complete. The catheter is then removed, and the incision site is closed by applying placing pressure at the puncture site for about 15 minutes or by using a closure device that seals the puncture site in the artery.

For several hours, this area will be checked periodically for bleeding and your blood pressure and heart rate will be monitored. In most cases, you will be required to stay in bed for a few hours and will be allowed to go home the next day. (For further information regarding what you will feel during the procedure, see the subsection "What Will I Feel?" in the section "Catheter Angiography" in Chapter 8, p. 171).

Tumor Embolization

A specific form of embolization is used to treat tumors. During this procedure, a catheter is maneuvered under fluoroscopic control to the major artery supplying blood to a malignant tumor so that the tumor can be selectively treated. Once the catheter is positioned at the tumor, several possible treatments may be delivered.

Tumor embolization is most commonly used in patients with primary malignant tumors of the liver (hepatocellular carcinoma) or tumors that have metastasized (spread) to the liver from another organ. The reason is that the liver has a dual blood supply: the hepatic artery and the portal vein. Although most blood reaches the liver through the portal vein, liver tumors usually receive their blood supply exclusively through the hepatic artery. Therefore, treatment agents injected directly into the hepatic artery can attack the cancer without harming most of the healthy liver tissue. Blocking the hepatic artery makes it possible to subject the cancer to a prolonged dose of a high concentration of the chemotherapy agent while the normal liver continues to receive blood supply through the portal vein. A small, isolated tumor can be treated with chemoembolization alone. Patients with large or multiple tumors may also receive radiation therapy, radiofrequency ablation (see below), or surgery.

Possible catheter-directed tumor treatments include:

1. Chemoembolization—injection of a high dose of anticancer medication directly into the artery supplying a tumor
2. Bland embolization—selective injection of small particles directly into the tumor arteries to suffocate the tumor, depriving it of oxygen and nutrients
3. Radioembolization—direct injection into the tumor arteries of radioactive particles that selectively irradiate the tumor(s). This procedure requires pre-radiation planning steps to ensure that the radioactivity is limited to the tumor. In some cases, other vessels may need to be selectively closed off to limit the radiation dose to normal tissues.

Chemoembolization

A variant of the embolization procedure is chemoembolization, in which a catheter is maneuvered under fluoroscopic control to the major artery supplying blood to a malignant tumor so that a high dose of anticancer medication can be injected directly into it. As part of the procedure, clot-inducing substances are introduced to block the artery. This cuts the blood supply to the tumor, preventing it from getting the nutrients and oxygen that it needs to grow. At the same time, it prevents the chemotherapy agent from being washed out by continuous blood flow.

The procedure usually takes about 90 minutes. You will be asked to remain in bed in the recovery room for 6–8 hours and in the hospital for up to 2 days.

After tumor embolization, many patients develop a *postembolization syndrome*, which consists of pain, fever, fatigue, loss of appetite, and nausea or vomiting. It represents the reaction of the body to breakdown products from the tumor. The pain, which results from cutting off the blood supply to the treated area, can usually be controlled with over-the-counter medications; IV drugs are sometimes required. It is normal to have a fever for up to 1 week following the procedure, and you will be given oral antibiotics. Fatigue and loss of appetite are also common and may persist for 2 weeks or longer. If your pain suddenly becomes worse or you develop a high fever, call your physician immediately.

You will be asked to return to the radiology facility for a follow-up CT or MRI scan every 3 months after tumor embolization to determine whether the cancer has shrunk and if any new tumors have developed. In about two-thirds of cases, tumor embolization can stop liver tumors from growing or even cause them to become smaller. This is important since it may preserve liver function and allow a relatively normal quality of life. The effect of the procedure generally lasts for about 10–14 months. Tumor embolization can be repeated if the cancer begins to grow or a new mass appears, as long as you are still healthy enough to tolerate the procedure and there is no technical factor preventing it.

Remember that tumor embolization is a palliative treatment for cancer and not a cure. It also may result in serious liver complications in up to 5% of patients and fatal liver failure in about 1 in 100 cases.

Uterine Artery Embolization
Uterine artery embolization is an interventional procedure to treat fibroids (myomas), benign tumors that arise from the muscular wall of the uterus. Although fibroids rarely become malignant, they may cause heavy menstrual bleeding, pelvic pain, and pressure on the bladder or bowel. The purpose of uterine artery embolization is to inject small particles (such as the ones described above) that block blood flow to the fibroids and cause the tumors to degenerate and decrease in size. Up to 90% of women with

fibroids report significant or complete resolution of their symptoms follow-ing the procedure. Typically, fibroids shrink to half of their original volume (20% reduction in diameter). Initial follow-up studies show that treated fibroids rarely grow back and that it is unusual for new fibroids to develop in the uterus after the procedure.

Under fluoroscopic guidance in the interventional radiology suite, a cath-eter is introduced into each groin and maneuvered into the uterine artery on the side opposite the puncture. Contrast is injected to make certain that the catheters are properly positioned and to provide a road map of the blood supply of the uterus and the fibroids. When the small embolic particles are slowly injected (on one side at a time), they tend to flow to the highly vas-cular fibroids and wedge in small vessels within the tumor. Within several minutes, this results in nearly complete blockage of blood flow (Fig. 9-6). Another contrast injection is performed to verify that flow to the fibroids is blocked, though there will still be some arterial flow to the normal parts of the uterus. The entire procedure takes about 60–90 minutes. In most cases, you will remain in the hospital overnight for observation.

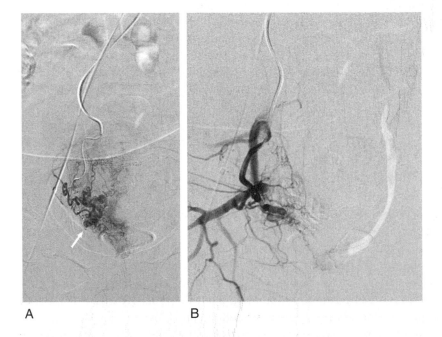

A   B

Figure 9-6. Uterine artery embolization. (Left) Selective contrast injection of the right uterine artery demonstrates diffuse contrast filling (blush) of multiple uterine fibroids (arrow). (Right). Post-embolization contrast study obtained after injecting 500 micron particles into the uterine artery shows occlusion of blood flow to the fibroids.

Most women have moderate to severe pain and cramping after the procedure, which can persist for several days and be controlled by medication. Nausea, low-grade fever, and fatigue are common and are related to the reaction of the body to breakdown products from the fibroid. You probably will be able to perform normal activities within 1–2 weeks. Normal menstrual cycles usually resume after the procedure. It is common for the amount of bleeding to initially be much less than before the procedure and then to increase slowly to a new level that is still much lower than before the embolization.

Complications of uterine artery embolization are infrequent. Less than 3% of women will pass small pieces of fibroid tissue, primarily if their tumor was located near the inner lining of the uterus and has partially detached. This may require a dilatation and curettage (D & C) to make certain that all of the fibroid material is removed from the uterus and to prevent any subsequent bleeding or infection. Occasionally, the embolization procedure may injure the uterus and make it necessary for this organ to be removed.

Most women undergoing uterine artery embolization have finished with childbearing. Although some women have delivered healthy babies after the procedure, it is not known whether uterine artery embolization decreases the likelihood of becoming pregnant. Therefore, many physicians recommend that a woman who wants to have more children consider surgical removal of individual fibroid tumors instead. Because of possible weakening of the uterine wall related to uterine artery embolization, women in the childbearing years are generally urged to use contraception for 6 months after the procedure and to undergo a cesarean section during delivery rather than risk the possibility of rupturing the wall of the uterus during labor contractions.

Thrombolysis

Thrombolysis is a procedure in which a medication is introduced through a catheter to dissolve abnormal blood clots and improve blood flow (Fig. 9-7). Blood clots that form within an artery or vein may continue to grow until they have completely blocked that vessel and caused severe damage to the tissues it supplies, including loss of an organ or extremity and even a fatal outcome. Blood clots also can break off and embolize to other sites in the body, often leading to serious complications.

Interventional thrombolysis is used to treat blood clots in various arteries and veins throughout the body. In atherosclerotic disease, clots may develop in severely narrowed arteries leading to the brain, heart, and extremities. Blood clots in the major veins returning blood flow from the extremities to

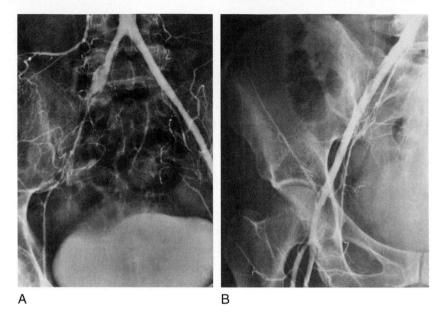

A   B

Figure 9-7. Thrombolytic therapy of acute arterial occlusion. (A) After angioplasty of the right external iliac artery, there was loss of the femoral pulse. Repeat arteriogram from the left femoral approach shows complete occlusion of the right external iliac artery at its origin. (B) After 8 hours of thrombolytic therapy, an arteriogram demonstrates lysis of the thrombus and reestablishment of the lumen. One year later, the patient had a normal femoral pulse and a patent artery.

the heart and lungs may either grow so large that they block venous flow or break off and flow to the lung, where they can cause a potentially fatal pulmonary embolus. Blood clots can also block the portal vein supplying the liver or obstruct fistulas or grafts that are needed for life-saving kidney dialysis.

The thrombolytic agent for dissolving the clot is introduced through a catheter that is inserted through the skin into the groin or arm and maneuvered under fluoroscopic guidance into the clotted vessel. The catheter is connected to a special machine that delivers the thrombolytic agent at a precise rate. Although most clots dissolve within 24 hours, at times it may take up to 3 days to completely remove the clot and restore blood flow. During this time, you will be closely monitored by the nursing and medical staff. An alternative procedure is to position a mechanical device at the site to physically break up the clot. This is a relatively quick procedure, lasting for less than 1 hour, and usually does not require a lengthy hospital stay.

At the end of the procedure, the catheter will be removed and either pressure will be applied to the puncture site to stop the bleeding or a closure device will be used to seal off the puncture site. For several hours, this area will be checked periodically for bleeding and your blood pressure and heart rate will be monitored. In most cases, you will be required to stay in bed for a few hours and will be allowed to go home the next day. (For further information regarding what you will feel during the procedure, see the subsection "What Will I Feel?" in the section "Catheter Angiography" in Chapter 8, p. 171.)

Thrombolytic therapy is an effective nonsurgical way of restoring blood flow that has been blocked by a clot. However, it cannot be used if for some reason the catheter tip cannot be maneuvered to the site of obstruction. Moreover, removal of the clot and renewed blood flow cannot repair damage to organs and tissues irreversibly injured by lack of circulation. As with any anticoagulant therapy, there is always a slight risk that bleeding will occur elsewhere in the body. Postprocedure bleeding occurring in the head can have serious consequences.

Venous Access Procedures

In most cases, a simple IV line is sufficient for drawing blood or for giving medications or nutrients on a short-term basis. However, if there is a need for long-term venous access (weeks, months, or even years), a special catheter must be placed into a major vein (usually a large vein in the arm or neck) so that it can be accessed easily and often for a prolonged period. This catheter is maneuvered into a central vein near the heart so that blood can be repeatedly drawn, medications and nutrients continually given, and long-term renal dialysis performed without the discomfort and stress of multiple needle sticks. Central venous access is especially important when there is a need to deliver a large volume of an irritating solution (antibiotics, transfusions, IV feeding, and sclerosing chemotherapy agents) that would seriously damage smaller, more peripheral veins and cause local tissue damage if it leaked out of the vein.

The major indications for interventional venous access procedures are:

- Long-term IV antibiotic therapy
- Chemotherapy for cancer
- Long-term IV feeding (total parenteral nutrition, or TPN)
- Hemodialysis for kidney failure (transfer of blood from the body to a special machine that removes wastes and extra fluid and then returns the cleansed blood to the patient)

Some central catheters may be inserted at the bedside without imaging guidance. One example is the peripherally inserted central catheter (PICC)

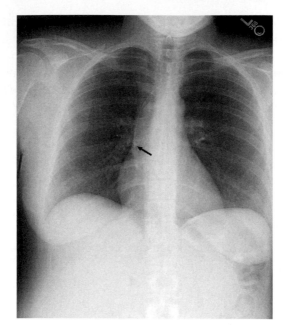

Figure 9-8. PICC line. The tip of the catheter (arrow) lies in the proper position in the lower part of the superior vena cava.

line, which is inserted into a vein near the elbow and threaded through the upper arm and eventually into the superior vena cava, the large vein that drains blood from the upper extremities into the heart (Fig. 9-8). Other central catheters are introduced with ultrasound guidance into the jugular veins in the neck, the subclavian veins just under the clavicles, or the femoral veins in the groin. The position of a PICC line is confirmed by a chest radiograph to make certain that the tip is not in an incorrect position (too high, too low, or heading upward into the neck). Similarly, a chest radiograph is obtained after jugular or subclavian catheter insertion to check its position and identify complications.

For long-term venous access, a larger tunneled catheter is inserted under fluoroscopic guidance in the interventional radiology suite or occasionally in an operating room. The tunneled catheter has a cuff that stimulates the growth of tissue that holds the catheter securely in place. Some tunneled catheters are attached to a small reservoir that permits medication to be infused continually at a constant rate.

The placement of a venous catheter is a relatively quick procedure that lasts for less than 1 hour. Once the proper position has been confirmed, you may be allowed to go home and rest for the remainder of the day. You may resume your normal activities the next day, though you should avoid heavy lifting. If a tunneled catheter has been inserted, you may experience bruising, swelling, and tenderness in the chest, neck, or shoulder. Over-the-counter pain medications will help, and the symptoms should clear within a few days.

You will receive instructions on how to care for the site where the catheter was inserted and for your venous access device. You may be asked to flush the catheter periodically with a heparin solution to prevent the formation of blood clots, which could block the tip of the catheter.

Call your physician or other health care provider if:

- The catheter does not function properly
- There is bleeding or increased swelling at the insertion site
- There is redness, warmth, or fluid drainage at the catheter site or if you develop a fever (all signs of possible infection)

Inferior Vena Cava Filter Placement

The inferior vena cava (IVC) is a large vein in the abdomen that returns blood from the lower part of the body to the heart. In some individuals, large fragments of blood clots that have formed in veins of the leg and pelvis (deep vein thrombosis, or DVT) can break off and flow through the IVC to the lungs, where they can obstruct the pulmonary artery or one of its major branches (pulmonary embolism). Although most of these fragments are small and quickly dissolved by the body, larger emboli can cause chest pain, difficult and rapid breathing, and a rapid heart rate. If left untreated, large pulmonary emboli can lead to respiratory failure, circulatory collapse, and sudden death.

Risk Factors for DVT

Some risk factors for deep venous thrombosis are immobilization, long airplane travel, some forms of hormonal contraception, cancer, blood disorders, and recent surgery.

Inferior vena cava filters are metallic devices that can be placed in the IVC to prevent large fragments of clots from pelvic and leg veins from traveling to the lungs and causing pulmonary emboli. Initially, all IVC filters were permanently implanted in place. Newer devices can be removed when the risk of pulmonary embolism has decreased (Fig. 9-9). This eliminates possible long-term complications of permanent IVC filters, such as venous occlusion and filter migration.

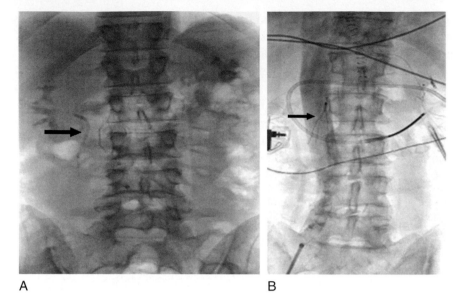

A   B

Figure 9-9. IVC filters. Spot images demonstrate the final positions of (A) a non-retrievable Trapease IVC filter and (B) a retrievable Celect IVC filter. Note the hook at the top of the filter on the right, which allows for future removal.

Inferior vena cava filters are placed when patients with DVT, which may embolize to the lungs, cannot be treated successfully by other means. These conditions include:

- Failure of anticoagulation (development of thrombi in pelvic and leg veins and pulmonary emboli despite treatment with blood-thinning agents)
- Contraindications to anticoagulation (patients at risk for pulmonary embolism who have another condition that increases the chance of bleeding, such as a gastric ulcer or a recent bleed into the brain, or who are about to undergo major surgery)
- Large clots in the pelvic veins or IVC
- High risk of pulmonary embolism, such as in trauma patients or those undergoing bariatric (weight-reduction) surgery

An IVC filter is placed under imaging guidance in an interventional radiology suite or occasionally in an operating room. A catheter inserted through the groin (or neck) is advanced to the IVC in the midabdomen. When the catheter is in the correct position, which may be verified by a small injection of contrast material, the filter is threaded through the catheter and released into the IVC, where it becomes attached to the wall of the blood vessel.

At the conclusion of the procedure, which usually takes about 1 hour, the catheter is removed and pressure is applied to the puncture site to stop any bleeding. After a short stay in the recovery room, where the puncture site will be checked periodically for bleeding and your blood pressure and heart rate monitored, you may be allowed to go home. If the filter was inserted through a vein in your groin, you should not drive for 24 hours or lift heavy objects or climb stairs for 48 hours. (For further information regarding what you will feel during the procedure, see the subsection "What Will I Feel?" in the section "Catheter Angiography" in Chapter 8, p. 171.)

An IVC filter can be removed by reversing the process. A special catheter is inserted through the groin (or neck) that grabs hold of the small hook or knob at one end of the filter. The filter is then slowly pulled to the puncture site and removed from the body.

In rare cases, an IVC filter can break loose from its attachment to the vein wall and travel to the heart or lungs, causing injury or even death. Another rare complication is that the filter becomes so filled with clots that it blocks blood flow in the IVC, causing swelling in both legs.

Nonvascular Procedures

Needle Aspiration Biopsy

Needle aspiration biopsy is an interventional diagnostic procedure, performed under imaging guidance, in which a thin, hollow needle is inserted into a nodule or mass to extract cells that, after being stained, are examined by a pathologist under the microscope (Fig. 9-10). This is especially important when a tissue diagnosis is needed to determine whether a mass is benign or malignant. If a mass is malignant, needle aspiration biopsy may permit a definitive diagnosis of the type of tumor, which can help guide the approach to treatment.

Needle aspiration biopsy is much safer and less traumatic than open surgical biopsy. Significant complications are rare and depend on the part of the body involved. Because only a small biopsy sample is obtained, there may be an insufficient number of cells to make a definitive diagnosis. Moreover, since relatively few cells are taken, the biopsy sample may fail to include the abnormal cells (sampling error) and produce a false-negative result.

There are two basic types of biopsy needles. A *fine* needle is thin, smaller than that used to take blood, and a syringe is used to withdraw fluid or clusters of cells. A *core* needle often has a cutting tip. Activation of an automated spring-loaded mechanism moves the outer sheath forward to cut a "core" of tissue and keep it within the needle trough. This procedure is usually repeated 3–6 times to obtain an adequate sample.

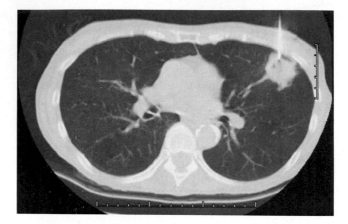

Figure 9-10. Needle aspiration biopsy. CT demonstrates the position of the biopsy needle in a lung nodule in the left lower lobe. Cells were sent to the laboratory for cytologic testing, and the results indicated that the mass represented an infiltrating, poorly differentiated adenocarcinoma.

During the biopsy procedure, you should remain as still as possible. You may be asked to hold your breath several times. Once the biopsy is completed, the needle is withdrawn, pressure is applied to stop any bleeding, and the puncture site is covered with a dressing. The procedure is usually completed within 1 hour, after which you will be taken to a recovery room and observed for several hours before being allowed to return home. For biopsy of a lung nodule, you will usually have a plain chest radiograph soon after the procedure to exclude the possibility of a pneumothorax (abnormal presence of air in the pleural cavity from leakage at the puncture site that may compress the lung and prevent it from fully expanding). Occasionally, this requires the insertion of a chest tube between the collapsed lung and the chest wall to remove the air and reexpand the lung.

You may experience soreness at the biopsy site as the effect of the local anesthetic fades, but this should not last long. During the day after a biopsy you should not engage in strenuous activity. On the second day, you may return to your normal activities.

Infrequent complications of needle aspiration biopsy are bleeding and infection. Following a lung biopsy, the development of sharp chest or shoulder pain on breathing, shortness of breath, or a rapid pulse rate may be signs of a collapsed lung related to pneumothorax. If you experience these symptoms, you should go to the nearest emergency room and contact your physician, since you may need to have a small tube inserted to drain the air from your chest cavity.

Fluid Aspiration and Drainage

Fluid aspiration and drainage is an interventional procedure in which a needle is placed into an abnormal fluid collection and some or all of the fluid is removed. In the chest, drainage may include large pleural effusions (known as *thoracentesis*), cysts, and infected fluid collections (empyemas) in the thoracic cavity around the lungs. In the abdomen, there may be drainage of an abscess (collection of pus) or of free fluid (ascites) in the abdominal cavity (a procedure called *paracentesis*) (Fig. 9-11). If a localized fluid collection is infected, the needle may be exchanged for a catheter (a small tube with multiple drainage holes), which continues to drain fluid into a bag for several days until the infection has cleared and the tube can be removed. Specialized tubes with valves sometimes are placed under the skin for intermittent, long-term drainage.

Ultrasound or CT images are used to localize precisely the fluid collection and adjacent organs so that the radiologist can plan the safest course of the needle and avoid puncturing any important structure. The actual placement of the needle for fluid aspiration and drainage is also performed under imaging guidance. If you have had an abscess drained, follow-up scans are obtained to make certain that the entire fluid collection has disappeared. If you are an outpatient and have a drainage catheter inserted, you will be instructed in the care of the tube and bag and how to measure and document

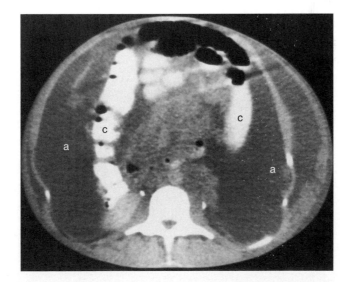

Figure 9-11. Ascites. CT scan through the lower abdomen shows a huge amount of low-density ascitic fluid (a), with medial displacement of the ascending and descending portions of the colon (c). This fluid was successfully drained by the radiologist.

the amount of drainage per day. You may also need to irrigate (*flush*) the catheter periodically to keep the drainage material from clogging the tube.

Tube Placement

Interventional radiologists insert a variety of tubes through the skin into organs in the abdomen. These include placement of:

- Gastrostomy tube—a feeding tube into the stomach or jejunum
- Cholecystostomy tube—placed into the gallbladder to remove infected bile in a patient with cholecystitis (inflammation of the gallbladder) who is too ill to undergo surgery
- Nephrostomy catheter—placed through the kidney into the collecting system to drain urine when its normal flow is obstructed (Fig. 9-12)
- Biliary stent—a catheter placed in the bile ducts to decompress the system and bypass an obstruction

In patients with end-stage liver disease, a transjugular intrahepatic porto-systemic shunt (TIPS) procedure can be performed to decrease portal hypertension (elevated pressure in the portal vein). This is a serious condition that can cause bleeding varices, severe ascites (accumulation of a large amount of protein-rich fluid in the abdomen), and the Budd-Chiari syndrome (blockage of one or more of the veins that return blood from the liver to

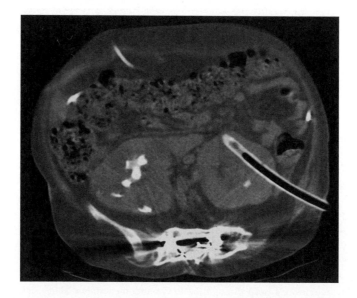

Figure 9-12. Nephrostomy tube. CT scan shows the nephrostomy tube, which was placed in the left renal pelvis to drain a urinary obstruction due to a renal stone.

the heart). A catheter inserted in the jugular vein in the neck is passed under fluoroscopic guidance to the liver and out into one of the hepatic veins. A needle that punctures the wall of the hepatic vein is advanced so that it enters the portal vein, and a stent is positioned between these two vessels. The TIPS procedure produces the same physiologic effects as a surgical shunt or bypass—dramatically reducing portal venous pressure and easing the previously mentioned complications of this condition—without the significant risks of major surgery.

Tumor Ablation (Radiofrequency Ablation, Cryoablation, Laser Ablation, or Microwave Ablation)

Several ablation procedures are available that destroy a tumor through the pinpoint delivery of heat or cold. The most common is radiofrequency ablation, a minimally invasive technique to treat cancer. A needle electrode is placed into a malignant tumor under imaging guidance. Then an electrical current in the range of radiofrequency waves is passed between the needle electrode and grounding pads placed on the patient's skin (usually the thigh or back). These currents create heat around the electrode, which is directed into the tumor to destroy the abnormal cancer cells. The intense heat from radiofrequency energy also causes small blood vessels to close, decreasing the risk of bleeding. The dead tumor cells are gradually replaced by scar tissue, which shrinks over time. Each radiofrequency ablation, which is sufficient to create an area of tumor destruction about 1–2 inches in size, takes about 15 minutes. In larger tumors, multiple ablations are performed. The entire procedure is usually completed within 1–3 hours.

Radiofrequency ablation is most commonly employed to treat hepatocellular carcinoma, a primary liver cancer that tends to be slow-growing and enclosed within a capsule. It also can be used to treat metastases to the liver, especially from colon cancer. Radiofrequency ablation is a good treatment option for small cancers (less than 1.5 inches in diameter) that are few in number in patients who:

- Cannot undergo surgery because of some other medical condition that would make an operative procedure very risky
- Have a liver tumor that would be difficult to reach surgically or would not have enough liver tissue left for the organ to function sufficiently after surgical removal of a tumor
- Have a liver tumor that has failed to respond to chemotherapy or that has recurred after surgical removal
- Have multiple small liver tumors that are too spread out to be removed surgically. Radiofrequency ablation may be combined with surgery to

treat a patient with several tumors in different locations. Unlike surgical removal, radiofrequency ablation can easily be repeated if a new tumor appears.

Radiofrequency ablation is also used to treat patients with early-stage primary lung cancer or with a small number of pulmonary metastases. This technique also can ease the pain of a tumor that has invaded the chest wall.

Immediately following radiofrequency ablation, you may experience pain that can be controlled by injected or IV medication. After the initial period, any residual pain can be eased by oral over-the-counter medicines. If you have a lung ablation, a chest radiograph will be performed to see if you have developed a pneumothorax (due to air leaking out of the lung at the puncture site), a complication that occurs in about 30% of patients. However, only about one-third of these patients need to have a chest tube inserted between the collapsed lung and the chest wall to remove the air and reexpand the lung.

About one in four patients develops a *postablation syndrome*, with flu-like symptoms that appear 3–5 days after the procedure and usually last for about 5 days. Infection and bleeding are very rare complications. Pain that persists for more than a week is uncommon.

Vertebroplasty/Kyphoplasty

Vertebroplasty is an interventional procedure used to treat a painful compression fracture of a spinal vertebra, which may be related to osteoporosis, trauma, or a malignant tumor. In most cases, it is recommended only after simpler treatments such as bed rest, a back brace, or pain medications have failed. The procedure also may be performed when pain medications cause side effects or in younger patients whose osteoporosis is related to long-term steroid use or a metabolic disorder. Vertebroplasty is not used for patients whose back pain is due to a herniated disk or arthritis or as a method to prevent fractures in patients with known osteoporosis. Kyphoplasty is a similar procedure that may be used to treat compression fractures in the lower half of the spine. However, it also has the potential to restore vertebral body height and reverse spinal deformities.

Vertebroplasty is most effective if performed on fractures that are less than 6 months old. The procedure consists of placing a hollow needle (trocar) through the spinal muscles and into the fractured vertebra under fluoroscopic guidance. When the needle is in the proper position, a special orthopedic cement mixture containing toothpaste-like polymethylmethacrylate is injected directly into small holes in the weakened spinal vertebra. This strengthens the bone, makes it less likely to fracture again, and provides pain relief.

In kyphoplasty, the initial step is to insert a balloon through the trocar into the fractured vertebra and then inflate it so that the bone is expanded as much as possible to its original height and shape. After the balloon is deflated and removed, a cement mixture is injected to fill the cavity made by the balloon (Fig. 9-13). This procedure is most effective if performed on compression fractures less than 2–3 months old.

These procedures are usually completed within 1 hour, though they may take longer if more than one compressed vertebra is treated. You will be asked to lie on your back for another 2 hours or so while the cement hardens.

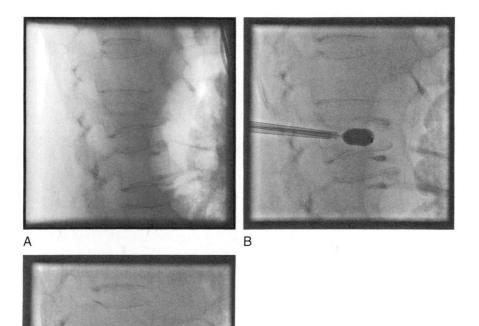

Figure 9-13. Kyphoplasty. (A) Initial lateral image of the spine shows a vertebral compression fracture. (B) On this view, a balloon has been inflated within the fractured vertebra. (C) After the balloon has been deflated and removed, a cement mixture is injected to fill the cavity made by the balloon. Although still compressed, the vertebral body is now closer to its original height and shape.

Then you are free to return home. You may be hospitalized overnight if you are especially frail, live far away, or have no one to take care of you at home. Most physicians recommend bed rest for the first day after the procedure, though you may get up to use the bathroom. You can then resume your normal activities, though you should avoid heavy lifting and strenuous exercise for at least 6 weeks.

Most patients experience significant pain relief within a few days. Many can return to their previous level of normal activity without the need for physical therapy or other methods of rehabilitation. Patients who have been confined to bed may be able to get up and resume some activities, thereby increasing muscle strength, improving mobility, and decreasing the risk of developing pneumonia.

The results of these procedures can be assessed on plain radiographs of the spine, since the cement mixture contains some barium powder that appears white on the images. With kyphoplasty, this permits an evaluation of the initial increase in the height of the previously compressed vertebral body, as well as long-term follow-up to determine whether there has been any new collapse.

Informed Consent

Whether to undergo a diagnostic or therapeutic procedure is a joint decision between the physician and a patient who possesses enough information to make an intelligent choice. In the absence of a serious emergency, a radiologist must obtain informed consent before performing any procedure with a significant incidence of serious complications. Virtually everyone agrees that this applies to all interventional procedures. However, there is no clear policy for less invasive studies, such as examinations requiring the IV injection of iodinated contrast material. Many radiologists inform patients undergoing contrast studies of the small but real risk of a potentially serious reaction. This is especially true if pretest screening has identified risk factors for a contrast reaction or if the patient has poor kidney function, conditions in which there is an increased risk of an immediate or delayed adverse reaction to contrast material.

What Should Be Disclosed?

For procedures requiring informed consent, it is generally accepted that the radiologist should explain the following in understandable terms:

- The diagnosis and nature of the condition or illness calling for medical intervention

- The nature and purpose of the proposed procedure (benefits)
- The known material risks and potential complications
- The relative probability of success for the treatment or procedure
- All available reasonable and acceptable alternatives to the procedure (including their materials risks and potential complications)
- The probable outcome if no procedure or treatment is performed

What are *material risks*? In general, you should be made aware of those risks that have the most severe consequences and have a substantial probability of occurring. All information must be presented in language that you can clearly understand. An explanation in highly technical and incomprehensible terms does not constitute true informed consent. If you do not speak English, a translator will be provided for you.

For interventional therapeutic procedures, it is important that you receive a realistic estimate of the likelihood of success from the proposed treatment, as well as the alternative treatments and the probable outcome of no treatment. It is important for you to realize that the hoped-for benefits of the procedure are not meant as a promise or a guarantee. You should also be informed about what to do if there is a complication. At times, this may merely be a reminder to consult your treating physician (or go to the emergency room or urgent care center) immediately if there is a complication, such as clearly described signs of postprocedure infection.

As part of the informed consent process, some radiologists supplement their explanations with educational material such as booklets and videotapes.

Who Must Disclose?

The radiologist who is to perform the procedure has the ultimate responsibility for obtaining informed consent. However, the radiologist may delegate this authority to your private physician or another doctor.

Withdrawal/Refusal of Consent

A competent patient has the right to withdraw consent at any time and for any reason. Once you demand the cessation of a procedure for which you had previously given consent, the radiologist must comply with your request and terminate the procedure as soon as it is medically safe to do so.

Implied Consent

Consent is presumed to exist in medical emergencies unless the physician has reason to believe that consent would be refused. When unexpected emergency conditions arise during an interventional procedure, especially if they are life-threatening, implied consent may be found to extend to modifications of the procedure beyond the scope expressly authorized. Other situations in which implied consent is presumed include a minor child who requires urgent care, a comatose patient who needs immediate treatment, a mentally incompetent patient, unavailability of a legal guardian, and an intoxicated patient who temporarily lacks the capacity to reason and give consent. If time permits, however, the radiologist should wait and obtain consent for the additional procedure. For example, if you have consented to a peripheral arteriogram and this demonstrates a severely narrowed artery that can be treated with balloon dilatation, the radiologist should not proceed to an angioplasty without securing your additional consent.

Documentation of Consent

The radiologist will ask you to sign a printed form indicating that a discussion regarding informed consent has taken place and that you understand the procedure and the benefits and risks associated with it. For very-high-risk procedures, you may even be given a test of your knowledge about the proposed procedure or be asked to write your own consent form to document your level of understanding.

10

PEDIATRIC RADIOLOGY

Many of the imaging examinations described extensively in this book may also be performed on children. Although the reasons for the procedures and their overall interpretation are similar, the preparations may be different. For this reason, there is a need for a separate chapter on pediatric radiology to identify the key differences that accompany these examinations. Furthermore, some imaging studies are performed almost exclusively in children. Infants and young children may be wrapped tightly in a blanket or restrained with sandbags or pads positioned on their sides to help them lie still during imaging.

Barium Studies

Various types of barium studies (such as upper GI series and barium enemas) using fluoroscopy are also performed in children. Dress your child comfortably in clothes that are easily removable. Your child will be given a gown to change into for the procedure. Avoid dressing your child in clothing with snaps or zippers, which could cause a confusing appearance on the radiographs, in case your child does not have to be completely undressed.

Parents usually may accompany the child into the examination room and remain throughout the study as long as they wear a lead apron to protect them from radiation. Women who are pregnant or may be pregnant will be asked to leave the examination room during the procedure. Please make sure that someone else is available to accompany the child during the study if needed.

The major difference between pediatric and adult examinations is the preparation prior to the study. An upper GI series must be done on an empty stomach. This means that your child cannot have anything to eat or drink by mouth or tube before the examination, for a period of time depending on his or her age. The times are as follows:

- 0 to 6 months: 3 hours
- 7 months to 2 years: 4 hours
- 3 years and older: 6 hours

You may want to bring a snack or drink for your child to have after the examination.

For a barium enema, there are different preparations according to the age of your child and the diagnosis or reason for the examination. Please pay close attention to the instructions. If the barium enema is being performed to evaluate for Hirschsprung's disease or constipation, there are no special preparations.

Voiding Cystourethrogram (VCUG)

A pediatric VCUG is a fluoroscopic examination of a child's bladder and lower urinary tract. It is often recommended to check for vesicoureteral reflux, a condition in which urine in the bladder flows upward back to the kidneys and can lead to an infection.

For this procedure, your child needs to lie on the x-ray table with the legs in a "frog" position. The radiologist will clean the urethral area with several cotton balls soaked in an iodine-based cleaning agent. The soap may feel a bit cool. Once the area is cleaned, a tiny feeding tube or catheter is placed in the bladder. Your child may feel some pressure and the sensation or urge to urinate. Once the catheter is placed, the tube is secured to your child's leg with tape. The catheter is then connected to a bottle of iodinated contrast material, which flows through the urinary catheter into the bladder. The radiologist then pulls the fluoroscope machine over your child and takes several x-ray images. Your child will be told to roll from side to side periodically and asked to hold the contrast in, even though he or she may feel the urge to urinate. Once the bladder is full, the radiologist will ask your child to urinate while still on the table. Small children and infants generally urinate on their own. If your child has difficulty urinating, sprinkling warm water on the abdomen typically provides sufficient stimulus. Once your child starts to urinate, more x-ray images are taken (Fig. 10-1). While your child is urinating, the catheter slides out without your child feeling any discomfort. When the bladder is empty, a few additional x-ray images are obtained to complete the study. The entire procedure, including the preparation process, takes an average of 20–30 minutes.

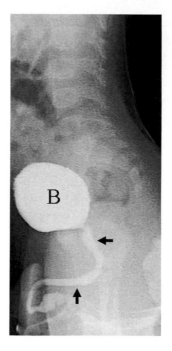

Figure 10-1. VCUG. Lateral view of the lower abdomen of a young boy shows contrast material filling the urinary bladder (B) and the urethra (arrows).

As with all imaging examinations using iodinated contrast material, always inform your physician of any medications your child is taking and if he or she has any allergies, especially to contrast materials, iodine, or seafood.

Ultrasound

This examination uses high-frequency sound waves to produce images of organs and soft tissues inside the body. With your child lying on his or her back on an examining table, the radiologist or sonographer spreads warm gel on the skin and then presses the transducer firmly against the area of concern, moving it back and forth until the desired images are obtained. Scanning over an area of tenderness may cause your child to feel pressure or minor pain. Once the imaging is complete, the gel is wiped off your child's skin.

If a Doppler ultrasound study is performed, your child may hear pulse-like sounds that change in pitch as the blood flow is monitored and measured.

The preparation for an ultrasound examination depends on the age of your child and the part of the body being examined. For an abdominal ultrasound, your child should have nothing to eat or drink for the following amounts of time:

- Infants: 2 to 3 hours
- 1 to 4 years of age: 3 to 4 hours
- 5 to 10 years of age: 5 to 6 hours
- 11 years and older: 8 hours

There are no food restrictions prior to a renal or pelvic ultrasound. Indeed, drinking liquids is required, since your child must have a full bladder in order for these studies to be performed. No special preparations are needed for ultrasound examinations of the spine, thyroid, neck, soft tissues, brain, or scrotum.

Computed Tomography (CT)

There are different preparations, depending on the type of CT scan that your child's physician has ordered. No special preparation is needed if your child is not being sedated or receiving contrast material. If your child is being sedated, you will be given specific guidelines to follow. For a CT scan of the abdomen or pelvis with contrast material, your child may be asked to drink one or two cups of a dilute barium mixture immediately before the procedure. This fills the intestines and makes it easier for the radiologist to distinguish bowel loops from other adjacent structures. If your child is to receive IV contrast material, he or she will be asked to fast (no solids or liquids) for several hours before the examination.

As with all imaging examinations using iodinated contrast material, always inform your physician of any medications your child is taking and if he or she has any allergies, especially to contrast materials, iodine, or seafood.

Magnetic Resonance Imaging (MRI)

Magnetic resonance imaging uses a powerful magnetic field, radio waves, and a computer to produce detailed pictures of organs, soft tissues, bone, and virtually all other internal body structures. If your child is to receive contrast material, an IV line will be placed before he or she is taken into the MRI control room. There the technologist will explain the scan to both you and your child, and will repeat the safety screening process to make certain that neither of you have any metal objects on your body or in your clothing (see p. 102), since these must be removed prior to entering the scanner room. If your child has an implanted medical device, you should try to bring information about the name of the device and its composition, the manufacturer, and the date of placement.

The MRI scanning room may feel cold, so be prepared with layers of clothing as needed. You will be asked to sit in a chair located near the scanner and may bring reading materials into the room to occupy yourself. The technologist will help to position your child on the MRI table according to the type of scan requested. While many children are positioned on their backs, some scans require lying on the stomach or side, head first or feet first. Due to the noisiness of the scan, you and your child will be given ear plugs to help block out some of the noise. Once comfortable on the table, your child will be moved into the tunnel of the MRI scanner. Whether your child can see or talk to you will depend on his or her position.

After the technologist leaves the scanning room, the actual MR imaging begins. For each of several sequences, the MR scanner makes a series of loud noises, which may sound somewhat different every time.

There are different preparations, depending on the type of MRI scan that your child's physician has ordered. No special preparation is needed if your child is not being sedated or receiving contrast material. Because of the length of an MR examination, sedation is required for all children up to 8 years of age. If your child is being sedated, you will be given specific guidelines to follow. If your child is to receive IV contrast material, he or she will be asked to fast (no solids or liquids) for several hours before the examination.

11

MISCELLANEOUS STUDIES

Bone Density (DEXA) Scan

What Is a Bone Density Scan?

Bone density scanning is an x-ray study used to measure bone loss. Also known as *dual-energy x-ray absorptiometry* (DEXA) or *bone densitometry*, this procedure measures bone mineral density (BMD), which generally correlates with bone strength and its ability to bear weight. Most commonly performed on the lumbar spine and hips, DEXA scanning is used primarily to diagnose osteoporosis and monitor its treatment (Fig. 11-1). Osteoporosis is a gradual loss of calcium and other minerals that most often affects women after menopause and causes bones to become thinner, weaker, and more likely to fracture.

Although a DEXA scan is valuable in assessing an individual's risk for developing fractures, this is also influenced by age, body weight, history of prior fracture, family history of osteoporotic fractures, and such lifestyle choices as cigarette smoking and excessive alcohol consumption.

(It is important not to confuse a bone density [DEXA] scan with a bone scan [see p. 146], a nuclear medicine test in which a radioactive tracer is injected to detect fracture, infection, or tumor in a bone.)

Why Am I Having this Test?

Bone density (DEXA) scanning is currently the standard for measuring BMD and diagnosing osteoporosis. This test is recommended for all women over the age of 65. In addition, your physician may order a DEXA scan if

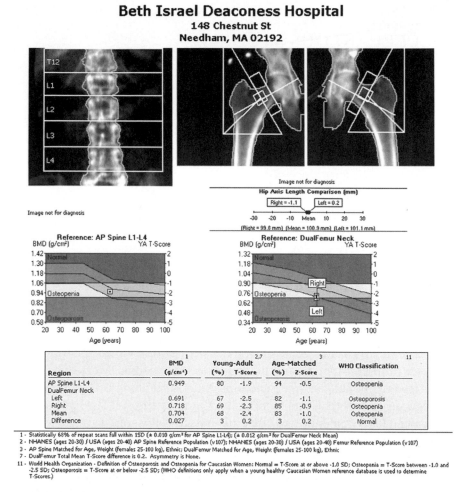

Figure 11-1. DEXA bone density results. The bone mineral density (BMD) values in this patient are consistent with osteopenia in both the lumbar spine and femoral necks.

you are a postmenopausal woman who has any of the following risk factors for developing osteoporosis:

- No use of hormone replacement therapy
- Personal or family history of hip fracture
- Low body weight or small body stature
- Cigarette smoking

Other potential risk factors for osteoporosis that may indicate the need for a DEXA scan include:

- Low physical activity
- Low calcium intake
- Excessive consumption of caffeine and alcohol
- Hyperthyroidism or hyperparathyroidism
- Use of medications known to cause bone loss (prolonged use of corti-costeroids [Prednisone], various antiseizure medications [Dilantin], or certain barbiturates)
- Diabetes, liver or kidney disease, or a family history of osteoporosis
- History of fracture after only mild trauma
- Plain radiographic evidence of vertebral fracture or other signs of osteoporosis
- Use of oral contraceptives (birth control pills)

Although DEXA scanning is usually performed in women, it may be ordered for a man with a clinical condition associated with bone loss.

Patients who have been treated for osteoporosis may undergo repeated DEXA scans to determine the effectiveness of this treatment. Some doctors recommend bone density studies every 1–2 years to monitor changes in BMD.

What Is BMD?

The World Health Organization has developed definitions for low bone mass (osteopenia) and osteoporosis. These definitions are based on a T-score, which compares the density of a patient's bone with that of a normal, healthy 30-year-old adult. A negative value indicates that you have thinner bones (lower bone density) that the average healthy 30-year-old; a positive value means that your bones are thicker and stronger.

The BMD is considered normal if the T-score is within 1 standard deviation of the normal young adult value. Thus, a T-score between 0 and –1.0 is considered a normal result. *Low bone mass*, or *osteopenia*, is the term for a T-score between –1.0 and –2.5 (Fig. 11-1). This signifies an increased fracture risk but it is not as serious as osteoporosis, which is defined as a T-score less than or equal to –2.5 (BMD more than 2.5 standard deviations below normal). Based on these criteria, it is estimated that 40% of all postmenopausal Caucasian women have osteopenia, and an additional 7% have osteoporosis.

In addition to the T-score, the computer generates a Z-score, which compares your BMD with that of others in your age group of the same size and gender. A negative value means that your bones are thinner (lower bone density) and weaker than those of most people in your age group; a positive value indicates that your bones are thicker and stronger. If the Z-score is unusually high or low, you may need to have further studies.

> Patients who have osteopenia in the lumbar spine or hip, the two regions usually measured with DEXA scanning, have a two to three times increased risk of suffering an osteoporotic fracture, not only in these areas but also elsewhere in the body. Those with a BMD in the osteoporosis range have about a five times increased risk of suffering an osteoporotic fracture.

What Should I Tell My Doctor?

Before going for a DEXA scan, make certain to tell your doctor if you:

- Are or suspect that you might be pregnant
- Have recently undergone a barium enema or have received IV contrast material for a CT scan or a radioactive tracer for a nuclear medicine scan. In either case, you will have to wait 10–14 days before having a DEXA scan.

Why Was the Bone Density Scan Developed and How Does It Work?

As a person ages, bone mass is naturally lost. The bones become thinner because existing bone is broken down faster than new bone is created. The lighter and less dense bones are weaker and more likely to fracture. Plain radiographs of the skeleton cannot detect mild bone loss. Therefore, DEXA scanning was developed to measure bone density precisely and provide a more accurate estimate of the likelihood that a person will someday experience an osteoporotic fracture.

A DEXA scanner sends a beam of low-dose x-rays with two different energy peaks through the bones being examined. The low-energy x-rays are absorbed primarily by soft tissue; the high-energy x-rays are absorbed by bone, with the amount varying with its thickness (bones that are strong and dense allow less of the x-ray beam to pass through them). The DEXA machine then subtracts the soft-tissue amount from the total to calculate the BMD and displays these results on a computer monitor.

How Do I Prepare for a DEXA Scan?

On the day of your scan, you may eat normally. However, you should not take calcium supplements for at least 24 hours before the examination.

What Does the Equipment Look Like?

A DEXA scanner consists of a large, flat table with an "arm" suspended overhead (Fig. 11-2).

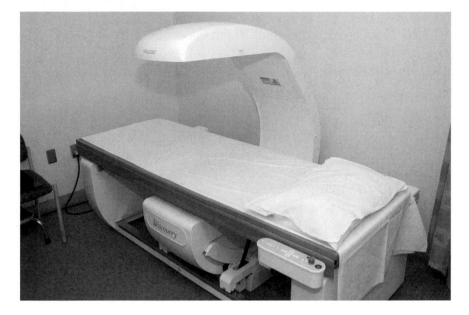

Figure 11-2. DEXA bone density machine.

How Is the Test Performed?

Bone density scans are unusually performed on an outpatient basis. For a study of your lumbar spine, you will lie on a padded table with your legs straight or with your lower legs supported on a padded box to flatten the pelvis and lower spine. For a study of your hips, your foot will be put into a brace that causes the hip to rotate inward. During the scan, the detector slowly passes over the area of interest, producing images on a computer monitor. It is important that you hold as still as possible. You may be asked to hold your breath for a few seconds while the x-ray picture is being taken so that the image is not blurred.

The entire bone density scan takes about 10–20 minutes to complete.

What Will I Feel?

Bone density scans are quick and painless. If you have back pain, it may be uncomfortable to lie still on the table during the scan.

What Are the Advantages and Disadvantages of a Bone Density Scan?

Advantages

- Most accurate technique for diagnosing osteoporosis and estimating the fracture risk

- Simple, quick, painless, and noninvasive
- Low radiation exposure (only about one-tenth of the dose of a plain chest radiograph)

Disadvantages

- Bone mineral density may be falsely elevated by lumbar spine abnormalities (scoliosis, previous surgery, arthritis, prior compression fracture) or a large amount of calcium in atherosclerotic arteries
- Can indicate the relative risk of an osteoporotic fracture but cannot predict who will suffer one
- Low BMD measurements may be caused by conditions other than osteoporosis, such as taking certain medications; hyperparathyroidism or hyperthyroidism; Cushing's syndrome (excess steroid production); premature menopause; vitamin D deficiency; and some cancers (such as multiple myeloma)

Treating osteoporosis

If your bone density is lower than normal, there are steps that can be taken to increase bone strength and thickness and reduce your risk of having a fracture. One alternative is to combine calcium and vitamin D supplements with weight-bearing exercise (such as walking) and weight training (such as lifting weights or using weight machines) plus medications such as calcitonin (Miacalcin), alendronate (Fosamax), or risedronate (Actonel). After menopause, women can use hormone replacement therapy to increase bone density, though there are side effects and contraindications to this treatment.

Hysterosalpingography

What Is a Hysterosalpingogram?

A hysterosalpingogram is an x-ray procedure that is usually performed in women who are having difficulty becoming pregnant (infertile) or have suffered several miscarriages. Filling the uterus and fallopian tubes with contrast material permits the radiologist to determine whether it flows normally back into the peritoneal cavity (Fig. 11-3) or if there is any narrowing or blockage that prevents the sperm from reaching and fertilizing an egg in the fallopian tube or any congenital abnormality, scarring, or mass in the uterus that prevents a fertilized egg from attaching to (implanting in) the uterine wall.

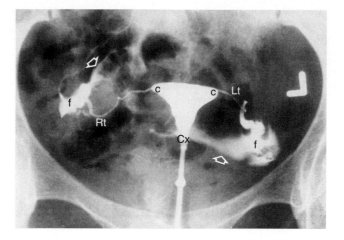

Figure 11-3. Normal hysterosalpingogram. The arrows point to bilateral spill of contrast material into the peritoneal cavity. Cx, internal cervical os; c, cornua of the uterus; f, fimbriated portion of fallopian tubes; Rt and Lt, right and left fallopian tubes.

Why Am I Having this Test?

Various abnormalities of the uterus and fallopian tubes can cause infertility and miscarriages. Your physician may order a hysterosalpingogam to search for:

- Blockage or severe narrowing of a fallopian tube due to scarring, which is most commonly caused by a prior infection (pelvic inflammatory disease, or PID) (Fig. 11-4)
- Abnormal shape or structure of the uterus related to a congenital condition or scarring (adhesions), or a mass such as a fibroid or polyp within the uterus that causes repeated miscarriages or painful menstrual periods

A hysterosalpingogram can also be performed to see whether a tubal ligation (sterilization procedure) to prevent pregnancy has been successful or whether the fallopian tube is again patent after a surgical procedure to reopen it.

What Should I Tell My Doctor?

Before going for a hysterosalpingogram, make certain to tell your doctor if you:

- Are or might be pregnant
- Currently have a pelvic infection (PID) or a sexually transmitted disease such as gonorrhea or *Chlamydia*

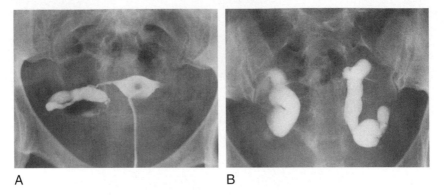

A   B

Figure 11-4. Hydrosalpinx. Examples of unilateral (A) and bilateral (B) gross dilatation of the fallopian tubes without evidence of free spill of contrast material into the peritoneal cavity.

- Know that you are allergic to iodine-containing contrast material
- Are allergic to foods containing iodine (such as shrimp and other shellfish)
- Have any bleeding problems or are taking a blood-thinning medicine such as aspirin or warfarin (Coumadin)
- Have diabetes or are taking metformin (Glucophage) for diabetes
- Have asthma, kidney or thyroid problems, or multiple myeloma

Why Was the Hysterosalpingogram Developed and How Does It Work?

Plain radiographs of the pelvis cannot demonstrate the internal structure of the uterus and fallopian tubes. Ultrasound can provide good images of the uterine cavity but is limited in demonstrating the fallopian tubes. The hysterosalpingogram using iodinated contrast material was developed to show whether there is an abnormality in either of these structures that could be preventing pregnancy or causing repeated miscarriages.

Historical vignette

Early hysterosalpingograms (1914) used Collargol, a colloidal silver preparation, but this caused severe irritation. Later, oxygen and oily iodine-containing materials were used to provide contrast. In the 1940s, radiologists began using less toxic water-soluble contrast agents for this procedure.

How Do I Prepare for a Hysterosalpingogram?

If you have regular periods, it is best to schedule a hysterosalpingogram during the week after your menstrual period has ended, at a time before ovulation, to make certain that you are not pregnant. The procedure should not be performed if you have an active pelvic inflammation or an untreated sexually transmitted disease. You will be asked to sign a consent form indicating that you understand the slight risks of a hysterosalpingogram and agree to have it performed.

On the night before the procedure, you may be asked to take a laxative or an enema to clean your bowel so that the uterus and fallopian tubes can be seen clearly. You also may be given an antibiotic to take before and/or after the examination to prevent any risk of infection.

What Does the Equipment Look Like?

The hysterosalpingogram is performed on standard x-ray equipment that is equipped with a fluoroscope, which enables the radiologist or technologist to follow the contrast material as it fills the uterus and then passes through the fallopian tubes before spilling out into the peritoneal cavity.

How Is the Test Performed?

A hysterosalpingogram is usually performed as an outpatient procedure. You will be asked to take off your clothes below the waist and given a light-weight gown to wear. You will empty your bladder and then lie on your back on the x-ray table with your knees bent or your feet raised and supported by stirrups, much like a pelvic examination. Prior to the procedure, you may be given a mild sedative to minimize any discomfort.

The radiologist will put a smooth, curved speculum (resembling a duck's bill) into your vagina. The size and shape of your uterus may be assessed by the radiologist, who will insert two fingers inside your vagina and press down on your lower abdomen with the other hand.

After the cervix is cleaned with an antibacterial soap, a stiff tube (cannula) or a bendable tube (catheter) is inserted through the cervix into the uterus. A thin clamp (tenaculum) may be placed on the cervix to hold it steady while the contrast material is introduced. After the speculum is removed, you will be carefully positioned under the fluoroscope. Contrast material is gently allowed to fill the uterine cavity. If the fallopian tubes are open, it will flow through them and spill into the peritoneal cavity, where it will be absorbed naturally by the body. Any abnormalities in the uterine cavity or fallopian tubes will be visible on a TV monitor. Fluoroscopic x-ray images are taken, and additional views may be obtained with you placed in a different position or with the examination table tilted. At times, you may be asked to rest on the table for up to 30 minutes so that delayed images can be obtained.

Once all of the images have been taken, the cannula or catheter is removed and you will be allowed to sit up and get dressed. You may immediately resume your normal activities, though you may be asked to refrain from intercourse for a few days. The entire procedure usually takes 15–30 minutes.

What Will I Feel?

You probably will experience some mild uterine cramping (like menstrual cramps) for the first few minutes after the contrast material is introduced. Some women have cramping that lasts for up to several hours. There also may be slight irritation of the peritoneum that causes mild generalized lower abdominal pain, but it does not last long. It is normal to experience vaginal spotting for a few days after the examination.

Call your doctor immediately if you have:

- Heavy vaginal bleeding (soak more than one tampon or pad in 1 hour)
- Fever
- Severe abdominal pain
- Vaginal bleeding that lasts for more than 3–4 days

What Are the Benefits and Risks of a Hysterosalpingogram?

Benefits

- Short, minimally invasive procedure with rare complications
- Can demonstrate abnormalities explaining the reason for infertility or repeated miscarriages
- Reported to occasionally open blocked fallopian tubes and allow a previously infertile woman to become pregnant

Risks

- Infrequent pelvic infection (<1%) that occurs primarily in women who have evidence of prior infection involving the fallopian tubes
- Rare puncture of the uterus or damage to the fallopian tubes
- Rare allergic reaction to iodine-containing contrast material

Glossary

Abscess. Encapsulated collection of pus.

Acoustic shadowing. Intensely echogenic line at the surface of a structure that blocks the passage of sound waves, indicating that there is fluid above it (such as the back wall of a cyst).

Adenocarcinoma. Malignancy of glandular tissue.

Adenoma. Benign neoplasm that grows in a gland-like structure.

Adenopathy. Enlargement of the lymphatic glands.

Adult respiratory distress syndrome (ARDS). Severe pulmonary congestion due to diffuse injury to the alveolar-capillary membrane.

Aneurysm. Sac formed by localized dilatation of the wall of a blood vessel.

Angiography. Invasive x-ray test in which contrast material is injected through a catheter inserted in the groin or arm to produce images of arteries and veins in various parts of the body.

Angioplasty. Interventional procedure to dilate a narrowed or blocked artery.

Anterior. Toward the front of the body.

Anticoagulant. Substance that suppresses or delays coagulation of the blood.

Ascites. Accumulation of fluid in the abdominal cavity.

Atherosclerosis. Progressive narrowing and hardening of the arteries over time; risk factors accelerating this process include high blood pressure, smoking, and diabetes.

Attenuation. The degree of whiteness on a CT scan.

Axial. Plane through the body that is parallel to the ground and separates superior (above) from inferior (below); also known as *transverse*.

Bariatric. Referring to weight-reduction surgery.

Benign. Tumors that closely resemble their cells of origin in structure and function and remain localized.

Calcification. Deposition of calcium salts in a tissue, which appears white on radiographs.

Carcinoma. Malignant neoplasm of epithelial cell origin.

Catheter. Thin plastic tube through which contrast material is injected to produce images of arteries and veins in various parts of the body.

Central nervous system (CNS). Consisting of the brain and spinal cord.

Cerebrospinal fluid (CSF). Clear, colorless fluid that fills the ventricles of the brain and the area around the spinal cord.

Cerebrovascular disease. Any process that is caused by an abnormality of the blood vessels or the blood supply to the brain.

Claudication. Pain in the legs with exercise due to decreased blood supply.

Congenital. Existing at birth.

Contrast material. Substance that is opaque to x-rays; when administered, it allows a radiologist to examine the organ or tissue it fills.

Coronal. Plane through the body that is perpendicular to the ground and separates the front (anterior) from the back; also known as *frontal*.

Coronary arteries. Vessels supplying blood to the heart muscle.

Cyst. Sac-like structure, usually filled with fluid.

Cytology. Microscopic examination to determine cell structure.

Density. Degree of whiteness on an image.

Dislocation. Displacement of a bone no longer in contact with its normal articulation at a joint.

Distal. Situated away from the point of origin or attachment (as of a limb or bone).

Diuretic. Substance or drug that tends to increase the amount of urine.

Dissection. Separation of layers of the wall (as in the aorta).

Echogenic. Producing a relatively strong reflection (white) in ultrasound.

Edema. Accumulation of abnormal amounts of fluid in the intercellular fluid tissue spaces or body cavities.

Effusion. Accumulation of fluid (as in the pleural or pericardial space).

Embolization. Interventional procedure to stop bleeding from an artery.

Embolus. Any foreign matter, such as a blood clot, carried in the bloodstream.

Endometrium/endometrial. The inner lining of the wall of the uterus.

Enhancement. Increased opacity (whiteness) of a tissue after the administration of contrast material.

Etiology. Cause of a disease.

Focal. Localized.

Fracture. Break in a bone.

Hematogenous. Spread by means of the bloodstream.

Hematoma. Hemorrhage trapped in body tissues.

Hemorrhage. Bleeding or abnormal blood flow from a vessel into tissue.

Hepatitis. Inflammatory disease of the liver.

Heterogeneous. Composed of materials that have different structures or qualities.

Homogeneous. Composed of material of similar or identical structure or quality.

Hyperlucency. Overly black appearance on a radiograph.

Hypertension. High blood pressure.

Iatrogenic. Resulting from the activity of diagnosis or treatment by medical personnel.

Idiopathic. Having an unknown cause for underlying disease.

Infarction. Death of tissue because of interruption of the normal blood supply.

Infiltrating. Spreading into surrounding tissue.

Inflammation. Initial response of body tissue to local injury.

Intraluminal. Within the empty space of a hollow viscus.

Intramural. Within the wall of an organ.

Ischemia. Lack of blood supply in an organ or tissue.

Isoechoic. Structures that have the same echogenicity.

Lateral. Side.

Lipoma. Tumor composed of fat.

Lumen. Inner open space or cavity of a tubular organ, such as a blood vessel or the intestine.

Lymphoma. Neoplastic disorder of lymphoid tissue.

Metastasis. Spread of disease to another organ or tissue in the body.

Mucosal. Referring to the inner lining of a viscus.

Multiple myeloma. Bone marrow malignancy.

Myocardial. Relating to the muscle of the heart.

Myocardial infarction. Infarction of the heart muscle.

Necrosis/necrotic. Relating to death or decay of tissue.

Neoplasm. New, abnormal growth, especially uncontrolled and progressive.

Opacity. An area of whiteness on an image.

Osteoarthritis. Degenerative changes in a joint.

Palpable. Able to be felt.

Parenchyma. Essential tissue of an organ.

Perfusion. Blood flow to an organ.

Pericardium. Membrane surrounding the heart.

Peripheral. Outside or away from the central portion of a structure.

Phalanx (phalanges). One of the small bones of the fingers and toes.

Pneumonia. Acute or chronic infectious disease of the lung.

Pneumoperitoneum. Presence of free gas in the peritoneal cavity.

Posterior. Toward the back of the body.

Prone. Lying with the front or face downward.

Proximal. Situated toward the point of origin or attachment (as of a limb or bone).

Pseudocyst. Pathologic collection of fluid that mimics a true cyst.

Pulmonary embolism. Blockage of the pulmonary artery or one of its branches by a blood clot from a vein in the leg or pelvis that breaks loose and travels (embolizes) to the arterial supply of one of the lungs.

Radiopaque. Appearing white on an x-ray image.

Renal. Referring to the kidney.

Sagittal. Plane through the body that is perpendicular to the ground and separates left from right; also known as *lateral*.

Sarcoma. Highly malignant tumor arising from connective tissues.

Signal intensity. The degree of whiteness on an MRI image.

Sonolucent. Producing no reflection (black) on ultrasound.

Stenosis. Narrowing.

Stress fracture. Fracture caused by repetitive stresses applied to the bone.

Stroke. Cerebrovascular accident; denotes a sudden and dramatic focal neurologic deficit.

Subdural hematoma. Collection of blood trapped between the dura (tough outermost meningeal covering of the brain) and the skull.

Superior mesenteric artery. Artery arising from the abdominal aorta that supplies the small bowel and some of the colon.

Supine. Lying on the back.

Symptoms. Subjective manifestations that the patient feels.

Teratoma. Neoplasm composed of various kinds of embryonic tissue.

Thrombolysis. Interventional procedure to dissolve a clot and reestablish blood flow.

Thrombus. Blood clot in the vascular system.

Transverse. Plane through the body that is parallel to the ground and separates superior (above) from inferior (below); also known as *axial*.

Ulceration. Destruction of tissue that creates an opening within a structure.

Vasculitis. Inflammation of a vessel.

Ventricle. Midline structures in the brain filled with cerebrospinal fluid.

Viscus. Any large internal organ, especially in the abdomen.

Index